SLEEP APNEA

Adjust Your Lifestyle to Deal With Insomnia

(How to Sleep Smarter & Increase Energy & Get
Help to Cure Stress)

Warren Lew

Published By Ryan Princeton

Warren Lewis

All Rights Reserved

*Sleep Apnea: Adjust Your Lifestyle to Deal With Insomnia
(How to Sleep Smarter & Increase Energy & Get Help to Cure
Stress)*

ISBN 978-1-77485-377-1

Legal & Disclaimer

The information contained in this book is not designed to replace or take the place of any form of medicine or professional medical advice. The information in this book has been provided for educational and entertainment purposes only.

The information contained in this book has been compiled from sources deemed reliable, and it is accurate to the best of the Author's knowledge; however, the Author cannot guarantee its accuracy and validity and cannot be held liable for any errors or omissions. Changes are periodically made to this book. You must consult your doctor or get professional medical advice before using any of the suggested remedies, techniques, or information in this book.

Upon using the information contained in this book, you agree to hold harmless the Author from and against any damages, costs, and expenses, including any legal fees potentially resulting from the application of any of the information provided by this guide. This disclaimer applies to any damages or injury caused by the use and application, whether directly or indirectly, of any advice or information presented, whether for breach of contract, tort, negligence, personal injury, criminal intent, or under any other cause of action.

You agree to accept all risks of using the information presented inside this book. You need to consult a professional medical practitioner in order to ensure you are both able and healthy enough to participate in this program.

TABLE OF CONTENTS

Introduction

A restful night's sleep is essential to an enjoyable quality of living. There are many benefits to the quality of our sleep. However, sleep quality is a factor that affects our productivity and , most important, our overall health.

Human beings can spend about three-quarters of their lives asleep. That's a lot of time when you consider it. We have evolved to require the time we spend sleeping because of the vital physiological processes that take place while we go to sleep. Our bodies use this opportunity to repair itself. Sleep can also boost memory.

Sleep deprivation affects us negatively. If we are sleeping for less time to make space for other activities it is causing harm to our bodies, and being at risk of accidents due to the lack of focus. A lot of accidents on the road result from drivers who fall asleep while driving or incapable of thinking quickly enough to prevent accidents due to lack of sleep. Performance at work and productivity at school are also affected when we're not getting an adequate night's rest.

In this guide, we'll explore some ways to achieve more restful sleep. These suggestions are taken from sleep experts and researchers who have taken the time to study the patterns of sleep and needs of humans. There is a growing concern among doctors that sleep does not receive the respect it deserves in the US. We're pushing people to work for longer hours and sleep fewer hours. Some executives say they rest for four hours. This can be harmful to their health overall and the damage that can be irreparable.

Chapter 1: Exercise

Exercise is one of the Natural Cure for Insomnia

If you're suffering from insomnia, there might be some solutions that can be done to ease the symptoms. However many of these solutions might be something we're not willing to try. For instance, one of the most effective ways to in getting a good night's sleep is to get regular exercise on a daily basis. While we all know that this is the case however, only a few will be motivated enough to put in the effort to tackle it. Is it something about exercising that makes it so hard to achieve? If exercise is an initial line of defence against sleeplessness, then why do we struggle to complete it?

It is necessary to exert effort from us regardless of how hard the exercise will be. If we're already feeling weak because of not sleeping well and this makes exercising seem harder. While this can result in a vicious circle of our lives, taking any discomfort that is temporary could make a big change in how you feel overall. The reason this happens is due to the fact that a small amount of exercise will release chemicals in the body which can help you fall asleep. In addition, it helps to restore the harmony in your body which could be out of balance because of the insomnia you experience.

It doesn't require you to be strenuous in order to be effective. In fact, the slightest amount of exercise several times a day, will make a huge difference in how you feel and the quality of you sleep. If it's too difficult for you to complete an entire workout at once, you can try engaging in a little exercise each when you eat. A 5 minute walk following your meal is likely create a dramatic change in this area.

In addition to releasing certain sleep-inducing chemicals to your body, it can also help you feel a general feeling of wellbeing. All of these could be a big help in helping you sleep at night and sleep until you're refreshed. Try a little exercises for a few weeks? You'll likely be amazed at the impact it could make on your life.

Chapter 2: Lifestyle and Treatments for Behavioral Problems

It has been stated numerous times in previous chapters that alterations to your lifestyle could help in treating insomnia and sleep issues. Here is what the doctors refer to as treatment for behavioral and lifestyle issues to assist you in getting better sleep.

Stimulus Control The bedroom must always encourage relaxation and sleep. Televisions and entertainment systems should not have a place in the bedroom.

The Sleep Restriction Treatment - Physicians suggest that you get up when you awake and lie in bed to go to sleep. A prolonged stay in bed for any reason other than sleep can aggravate the condition.

Cognitive Therapy is utilized to help with insomnia. The treatment involves the diagnosis of the root reason for the problem. The treatment provides patients with information regarding the effects of age-related changes on sleep as well as the sleep patterns and the effect of taking naps and exercising to ensure an enjoyable night's rest.

Relaxation Training - A variety of techniques can be taught to the patients such as PMR, for example. PMR (Progressive Muscle Relaxation method. PMR seeks to aid patients relax their major muscles. Other techniques include meditation, self-hypnosis and breathing techniques that are deep. Patients are encouraged to practice relaxation-training methods on a regular basis to guarantee that they are successful.

Sleep Hygiene is a consideration of the following elements that affect your lifestyle, habits, sleeping practices, and environmental influence. The four major areas sleep hygiene focuses on are your age, your internal biorhythm, emotional stresses that cause sleep problems and other substances such as nicotine, caffeine or alcohol.

The patterns of your sleep change as you reach 40. As you get older, nighttime awakenings are more frequent. These awakenings may affect your sleep quality. are able to get.

Your internal biological clock , or the circadian rhythm decides the amount of sleep you'll get.

Stressors that affect your mind are deadlines related to work or tests and school work which cause you to lose sleep in the time of night. Many people worry about what the day's plans are even though they're about to go to bed, which causes them to stay awake for long periods of time which causes sleeplessness.

If you consume caffeinated beverages before bedtime, you may not be able sleep off immediately. Nicotine also produces the same effect. Alcohol has the effect of sedating, sleeping you immediately however, it's quickly processed during sleep, which causes awakening at the end of the night.

The bedroom should be conducive to the quality of sleep. It must be quiet, cool and have little or none light. Patients are frequently recommended to hang thick curtains and use the earplugs and cover your eyes.

Chapter 3: Signs You're Not Inspiring a Good Night's Rest

Most most people are unaware of the fact that they're not getting enough rest. We believe that, since we got up, we've been through enough, continue doing our day-to-day things, and then comes night and we fall asleep. If we keep on the same pattern of not sleeping enough and waking up early, we're getting ourselves into greater problems. A lot of the symptoms of sleep loss aren't obvious. It is because we've repressed these symptoms and even forgot the satisfaction of having enjoyed a restful night's sleep. Let's look at some unexpected signs that indicate you're not sleeping enough. It's amazing to notice some or all of these every single day.

You'll need an alarm clock that will wake you up

If you've ever found yourself needing an alarm to get up at regular time, it means you're not sleeping enough Otherwise, your brain will get you up whenever you needed to. Our bodies aren't built to use an alarm clock to wake us up. For instance, during Saturday, we don't need an alarm clock. whyis that? It could be because we've rested enough. If you need to get up at a particular time, then go up early enough, and you'll be awake by that time.

You're angry and moody.

A lack of sleep can trigger anxiety and mood problems. This can lead to further issues in our health as well as social life if this is not addressed in a continuous manner. People will also be more prone to stress, anxiety, and depression. Experts in sleep have observed that this creates an unhealthy cycle, which causes us to be unable to fall asleep , even when we have some time to rest. Stress and anxiety are two of the most common causes of insomnia. They is often attributed to a lack of sleeping time in a short duration of.

Performance and productivity are not as high.

A lack of sleep can reduce our efficiency to a large degree. It causes a loss of focus and concentration, as well as the ability to solve the simplest of issues. A study conducted at the Harvard Medical School found out that sleeping disorders cost an American economic system $63 billion each year. This is because of the reduced productivity of the workers. The study also went on to conclude that it was not beneficial to remain up late at night working on projects and assignments since it adversely affected our performance the following day. We prefer to have an adequate night's sleep and perform optimally the following day. For students, the time of sleep is the time when our brains consolidate the day's learning and prepares for the following day's work by opening new pathways that help improve memory, creativity , and retention. Sleeping in a bad way can cause a decline in memory that will impact our performance.

Gain in weight

If you're not sleeping for longer hours, you could be losing weight. This might not be a definite indication, but there is an important connection between sleep patterns and eating habits. People who are less sleepy tend to become overweight or obese. The study was conducted at the Sleep and Chronobiology Laboratory of the Hospital of the University of Pennsylvania involved healthy adults to take part in a 2-week study of how sleeping restriction affected the way they eat. Half of the participants were required to remain awake until late at night while the rest rested for 10-12 hours. The people who stayed up until late ate 30 percent more calories, which led to an increase in weight. Researchers were astonished because they hadn't anticipated the results to be this large. Sleep deprivation can reduce the production of lepton, which is an appetite suppressing hormone that stimulates the production of ghrelin, which boosts appetite. With this information in mind I'm sure you'll desire to rest more. In addition, if you have more time to fall asleep after having your dinner and you're hungry, you could have a snack that isn't advised.

Low sexual libido

Insufficient sleep can influence your sex drive. If you notice your sexual desire decreasing it is a good idea to make sure you're sleeping enough. So in essence, less sleep means less sex. This is true for both males and women. The sleep experts have tried to clarify this by saying that those who sleep less tend to be extremely tired and not have time for sexual activity, are fatigued and experience an excessive amount of stress. In this attitude, having sex is the last thing they'd ever want to do.

It is easy to fall asleep as soon as you go to the bed

This is an unexpected indication that you're not getting enough rest. On average , it will take 15 minutes for you to go to sleep once you've settled in your mattress. If you notice that you fall to sleep immediately after lying down, you may be looking to extend the length of sleep you get.

You may feel sleepy throughout the day.

If you're feeling like you require a nap around 9 am, then you haven't had a decent night's rest. If you're snoring off during meetings or lectures even though they're boring, whatever they may be, then you're not getting enough rest.

Feeling emotionally tense

The lack of sleep can trigger your emotions into hyperdrive. An investigation has revealed that the brains of sleep-deprived individuals were 60% more sensitive to images that were disturbing or negative.

Insanity

People who are sleep deprived will have less precise and slower motor abilities. The lack of sleep affects the balance and reflexes, reduces the speed of reaction, and decreases depth perception.

Chapter 4: Tips to Create Your Bedroom A Restful Space For Sleep

Ideally, your entire home should be one where you can relax. But, we all realize that there will be an unrest of some sort around us. A loud neighbour, busy roadway or barking dogs could be distracting and create stress. A place to unwind and unwind is crucial. when you leave, you must be in a place which encourages rest.

Here are some fantastic ideas to create your bedroom your sanctuary of rest.

1)Choose top quality furniture: If you're choosing furnishings for the bedroom,, choose furniture that is comfortable and of high quality. When you enter an elite hotel, one of the things you will notice is the bed and the solid wood furniture. A room that is well-crafted will allow you to unwind. No one wants to be in a shaky, cheap bed.

2.) Bedding: If you have furniture that is of good quality, you must get it dressed with high-quality bedding. Select pillows that help your head stay in place because, after all, you'll be spending 8 hours per day on it! Take into consideration the way you sleep. If you prefer sleeping with your back to the side you'll require a bigger cushion than if you are sleeping with your back.

Your bedding ought to be softest and most luxurious that you can afford. The thread count refers to the number of threads per square inch of bedding. The more threads counted higher, the more comfortable the bedding. High-quality sheets feel more comfortable on your skin, and will last longer.

3.) Control the temperature: The body's temperatures drop as you go into a deep sleep. A cooler bedroom can assist you in falling asleep faster since it accelerates your cooling system. The ideal temperature should be between 60 to 65 degrees.

4.) Mattress 4) Mattress: Do you feel that hotels' beds more comfortable than yours? Your mattress could be falling short. The sagging of your mattress can impact the quality of your sleep and comfort. The lifespan of mattresses is between eight to ten years. Hence, replacing it is essential.

5) Take away electronic devices: Do you have a habit of spending hours in your bed playing video games, or watching television? Perhaps you're required to monitor your social media prior to when you go to bed, and also whenever you awake in the evening. It's not healthy for you! Research has proven that taking out any electronic devices from your bedroom could give you an extra one hour of rest each night. It could mean the difference between feeling tired in the morning and then being full of energy.

6.) The alarm clock. If, for example, you've taken all electronics out of your home, how will you feel when you awake? We are all prone to using our phones to wake us up with a call, but in actual an old-fashioned alarm clock is better for the quality of our sleep. There are models that can be digital however, they'll illuminate in the dark. Why not stick to the old-fashioned way and get an old-fashioned mechanical alarm clock?

7.) Design your room Color psychology isn't an exact science but there is a consensus that it is important to choose hues that provide a relaxing feeling. If you're trying to stay clear of the traditional pastel and beige shades select a color that can create an effect.

Light purple is a great way to feel relaxed while light brown provides an impression of security.

Don't be scared of patterns. Rugs as well as throws that add interest and color to your living space. Avoid clashing colors and neon colors. patterns to give a feeling of peace.

A study conducted by Travelodge found that rooms with paint colors of silver, blue, or green offered the most peaceful sleep for their guests.

8.) Aromatherapy: Aromas can relax us and promote sleep. Vanilla and lavender are both efficient and also teach our body to identify their smells with sleep. Aromatherapy at night will help prepare your body and your mind to get ready for sleep.

If you make use of an essential oil diffuser and a diffuser and essential oils, you will soon be adept in making the right scent to unwind with. Here are a few scents that will help in sleeping and allowing your mind completely.

* Lavender, Frankincense, and orange. Lavender is soothing and relaxing for emotional and physical balance. Frankincense was utilized for thousands of years to treat illnesses and can boost the mood and boosts mood. The essential oil of orange will help to enhance the

uplifting qualities of the blend and aid in the state of relaxation.

"Lavender," lime and chamomile: with lavender is a well-known ingredient. The essential oil lime is believed to help support the respiratory system, while the chamomile oil helps fight depression.

9.) The white noise A continuous background sound can help to get rid of loud sounds and annoying background noises. Anything that creates a continuous sound can be used to provide white noise, like a humidifier or fan for example. If you prefer to avoid gadgets, there is an audio track to stream through the two platforms: Spotify or Pandora.

10) Maintain it neat Clean it up and reduce stress levels. The bedroom should be furnished with furniture, a bed and some treasured photos and other accessories, and only that. The shoes and clothes you wear must be tucked away. There shouldn't be an office or desk in your bedroom. You are here to relax! Take a

look at your mattress. What's better than to lie down in fresh sheets and a sweet-smelling bedding? Keep your bedding fresh and tidy and increase your quality of sleeping. If you awake in the morning , you should make your bed prior to leaving to go to work. Research has shown that those who are able to make their beds early in the morning are 20 percent more likely to rest well. Your bedroom is where you can relax so feeling content will only aid in the sleep process.

Last tip: Intimacy and sleep are the two primary reasons that your bedroom ought to serve! You should not be doing any work, watching television or gaming simply sleep, and sexual pleasure! Construct your mind to accept this, and you'll be able to enjoy your personal space and how it affects you.

Chapter 5: Energy Drinks The Secret to Getting Your Sleep and sanity!

According to his blog the Dr. Michael J. Breus Psychotherapist in Clinical Practice as well as a Board Certified Sleep Specialist, has a cautionary note on energy drinks. "They do not anymore marketed to people who are athletes or seeking a mid-morning or mid-afternoon boost between meals.

"Energy drinks are a huge market, and they are a part of the lives of the majority of Americans including teenagers and young adults. But when they first came onto the market they were categorized as dietary supplements.' They are now an upgraded variant of pop like Coke On Crack (to put it mildly).

"There's an increasing trend to include warning labels on products with high levels of caffeine. Often, it's much more than coffee or Turkish coffee! Researchers have published information on these drinks with high octane levels, but the industry itself isn't keen to release any information on its products, or even accept warning labels.

"In the online article which summarized the recent controversy I was shocked to find that while the FDA regulates the caffeine content of soft drinks that are cola-based to seventy-one milligrams for 12 fluid ounces, there is there's no restriction of this magnitude for energy drinks. With the lack details on the labels and the absence of any regulation in the market, it's difficult to determine what's inside an energy drink.

"That was said, at a minimum, the names of a few of these drinks should give obvious: Monster, Rock star, Tab Energy, and the all-time favorite Red Bull. My top choice, however (at the very least in its the name) is or Fixx (as In Fixx) Fixx) and WiredX505, which has 505 milligrams caffeine. This is about double the amount of a robust Starbucks drip. Are you shaking?

How energy drinks affect your Sleep

"It's definitely true that drinks with energy can, and sometimes have a positive impact when utilized properly. However, they've become so commonplace that I'm worried people consume they don't know what they contain and whether these ingredients are appropriate for inclusion within the diet of a person. This isn't just of the coffee. A lot of these drinks provide an excessive amount of sugar that you'll need to look for another one shortly after you've had your first. What's that imply to a restful night's sleep? Many things.

"Many people are accustomed to monitoring their coffee consumption during the last hours of the day when they are aware that it could impact on their sleeping patterns at night. What about energy drinks? These energy drinks can do more than hinder sleep. They can make you feel stressed nervous, jittery, and exhausted all simultaneously. If you're addicted, now is the right moment to review your habits and reduce your intake.

"Some ideas for cutting down in energy drink consumption:

Instead of waking to a sugary energy drink, opt for an ordinary cup of black tea or an easy coffee Joe.

* Instead of having an energy drink for lunch, you can sip an iced, unsweetened tea or any other teas you like.

Get rid of the afternoon lull by snacking on a protein-rich food with a bit of carbs, like slices of turkey served on whole wheat crackers, or an ounce of nut butter or celery sticks. If you're looking for a caffeine boost, consider drinking green tea.

Avoid any source of caffeine after 4 p.m.

"All natural energy is abundant when you've had a good night's rest. Try it for a while, and observe how few cans of energy drinks and soda drinks you'll need.

You'll definitely get more sleep and lose weight, but you'll also shed some also. Who wouldn't want that?"

FAVORITE FOOD SOLUTIONS TO Sleep

Food is your most trusted companion in the search to get a restful night's sleep. The issue in insomnia can be that it could make you wake awake at night due to blood sugar levels are to a low. A proper amount of healthy fats and protein can aid in stabilizing blood sugar throughout the night, allowing the liver to let out stored sugar molecules in time to get a good night's rest. The normal production of neurotransmitters within your brain can produce an energizing effect in your body when you're eating the right food.

*The Montmorency cherries are a sour one. Most cherries we see in stores are dark red color but the hue of these are lighter. With more than six times the amount of Melatonin, these cherry are an excellent alternative to ordinary cherries. The best deal is when you can find concentrated cherry juice which will increase the amount of melatonin more. In the time of peak season it is possible to find exclusive cherries in fine food shops. Make sure to search in the section of frozen foods for Montmorency concentrated cherry juice.

* The seeds of pumpkin as well as the powder that is made from pumpkin seeds contain a high amount of amino acids tryptophan. The body utilizes this amino acid to create serotonin, the neurotransmitter that makes us feel good. Keep in mind that's our 'feel-good and relaxation hormone. Also, pumpkin seeds contain significant quantities of zinc that the brain utilizes for the conversion of tryptophan to serotonin. People who aren't able to rest or get up at night usually have low levels of serotonin levels. Take 1 cup of seeds and half of a cup powder (with applesauce or other nutritious carbohydrates) as the

carbohydrate permits the tryptophan to enter the brain in greater amounts.

The grape skin is among the strongest antioxidants, that contains melatonin, as well as other polyphenols that are anti-inflammatory. Try this Dr. Oz's Strawberry Smoothie 2 hours before bedtime will ensure you get your recommended dosage of the grape's skin. To reduce blood pressure and ease you prior to bed, this smoothie is packed with strawberries, which contain Melatonin, as well as bananas, which are packed with potassium and magnesium.

Blend the following ingredients together in the blender:

1 tbsp grape skin-based powder

1 cup of frozen strawberries

1 banana

4 cubes of ice

*The plant Avena sativa is an important cereal grain made into oatmeal. Traditional herbal medicine suggests that this nutrient-rich, relaxing plant is ideal for those who have a stressed nervous system. The advantage of breakfast of oatmeal on a daily routine is the fact that it assists your body to cope better with stress that lasts for a long time. You know, who did you know?

To bring tryptophan to the brain, which helps you sleep, you'll need melatonin as well as the complex cabs Oats contain both in abundance. Include a co-factor which aids in the process of helping serotonin be produced in the brain, vitamin B6 and you're definitely fashioning. I know I know, you're thinking"no," but this is meant intended for breakfast. However, if you're smart you'll add it to your bedtime snacks to help you feel content and relaxed. One thing to note about arthritis is that Certain cereal grains can make it worse. Do you have arthritis? Remove all cereal and bread for two weeks, then put one back. What are you feeling? Are you suffering?

Stop eating these foods. No difference? Take a bite!

Have you ever thought about the fact that the liver is responsible for balancing our blood sugar levels? If our blood sugar is like a rollercoaster, it can almost guarantee a night full of sleepiness or awakeness. Many people don't think of the dandelion as a food that induces sleep but it is a liver cleansing properties , which can lead to more sleep.

Chinese medicine has relied on dandelions, along with other plants, to regulate hormonal imbalances for women. They also help balance hormones during postmenopausal and perimenopausal cycles. There is a belief among the Chinese are of the opinion (as me too) that dandelion can help balance in the liver as well as nourish the yin which then improves the functioning of blood and fluids as well as hormone balance.

"Yeah But it's an herb, how can you cook it?" you might be asking. You can steam or boil the dandelion and then sauté it in organic olive oil and garlic. Some like me, simply consume them raw as a salad. Don't pick them out of your backyard where you've likely applied insecticides and fertilizers. It is possible to grow it on your own (like me) or purchase it from the internet or at a natural food market or farmer's market.

If you can, buy olive oil from an olive grower in your area or winery since the olive oil sold in the shelves is runcid. Olive oil has no value after six months. It has lost its value and taste. Middlemen who ship olive oil transport everything on a slow boat since it's less expensive and it takes about a year for it to arrive at our shores. Then it is stored in the warehouse until they are able to sell it to grocery stores and other retailers. Who can tell how long it's been sitting in their shelves? When you first taste fresh-made olive oil (it's as good as a wine) you'll not be able to stop!

EXERCISE

Do you want to have a more peaceful sleeping? Exercise! It helps release the essential chemical substances that you require to replenish your body. It also helps your body in all aspects of your life.

There are four kinds of exercises:

* Aerobic exercise like walking in the water, swimming or riding bikes will increase your heart rate and respiration to increase the health of your heart as well as your circulation system.

* Strength training builds muscles and prevent loss of muscle due to age.

* Stretching exercises help keep your body flexible and limber and allows you to move with greater ease of motion when you get older.

* Balance exercises strengthen leg muscles, reducing the risk of falling.

Do you want to get the maximum effect on your sleeping? Nothing can do that like exercising. Even a few moderate moves that are based on the suggestions above could transform your life for the better. Everybody should do it on a regular basis, if not every day adults, children and even senior citizens.

If you work an occupation that is sedentary, (like my job) an absence of physical activity could reduce how well you sleep (which did). Sleep is more than resting, it's about healing and repair. If you're not seeing anything happening the sleep cycle may become (and is) in a rut. Do you know it is the best time to be preparing for a restful night's rest? Morning.Taking the stairs or walking instead of riding in a car and such offers you additional options to get outside of your regular fitness routine to add activity to your day. However, it's the actual physical effort of swimming, running (what I am passionate about) and biking, lifting weights and the like which can lead to longer and better sleep.

Worse time to pull a Schwarzenegger? Bedtime. You might get tired by doing this however it also increases the heartbeat and stimulates your body , so you'll feel like Ms. Wide awake. If your job or your life requires you to exercise during the night and you are unable to stop it, do so about two hours prior to going to bed. This will allow your body time to cool and also give you the chance to replenish your water.

Perform some stretching before going to bed. It is best to do this every night in a slow and leisurely way will help prepare your body for sleep.

Take a deep breath. I lost my 26 year old sold son 12 years ago. Ever since that time, I must remind myself to breathe deeply. Actually, I hold my breath. My counselor for grief assures me that breathing is normal following an experience like this. Trust me when I say that the breathing issue has influenced my sleeping routine.

Numerous factors can contribute to insomnia such as stress, illness and even post-traumatic stress that is short-term. If you've lost the child you loved and you're not sure what to do regarding it. Have you experienced any events or changes bothering you or taking up your thoughts? In your mind, this problem could be disrupting your sleeping. As opposed to athletes, we can't breathe as in the way our bodies require to breathe. In order to breathe deeply it is necessary to use your abdominal, chest lower back, and ribcage. The benefit is that it aids in to relax. Relax with me in closing your eyes. then taking deep, slow breaths, each one more deep than the previous. In through your nose , and to exhale through the mouth.

Did you have the knowledge that progressive muscle relaxation is just as effective as stretch of muscles? Once you're lying down and comfortable, get on your feet and tense the muscles as tight as possible. Do a count to ten, and then let them relax. Repeat this exercise for each muscle group within your body, working up to the highest point of your head.

We'll go into more detail about exercise later on.

MEDITATION

White bread me is about to take you Asian on you yet again by offering you meditation. Instead of sitting in a secluded position trying to not think of any thoughts, we'll be using mantra, which is a word or phrase repeated repeatedly. In the Universe can be described as energy. Sound is also energy. Repetition of certain phrases or words repeatedly in your head or in public places us with the universal energy. It also counteracts thoughts that cause anxiety.

If you're anything like me and your brain doesn't want to shut down when you try to unwind for sleep Perhaps this is the solution for you. You can choose any word you want, however it's recommended to use positive phrases like joy, peace, love or any other word you feel is pleasant.

The advantage of a mantra is it doesn't cause any side effects as sleep medication. Meditation, mantras such as yoga, tai chi, and yoga all have the potential to soothe a disturbed mind and relieve tension. When you wake up in the early hours of the morning You can make use of these to return to sleep more quickly This is always a benefit.

A sequence of flowing, slow body movements, tai-chi is a practice that emphasizes relaxation, concentration and the conscious flow to the entire body of energy. If you've ever been in a public space and noticed an entire group of people moving in sync, you've observed tai chi. Why are you hanging in an outdoor space? Originated from martial arts, nowadays it's a method to calm your mind, strengthening the body and reducing stress. Focusing on breathing and focusing on the present.

It is safe for everyone of everyone of all ages and fitness levels including kids, seniors as well as those recovering from injuries. Tai Chi is similar to yoga. Once you've mastered the fundamentals, you can do it in a group or on your own. The benefit of mastering these techniques for relaxation are immense. Make them part of your evening routine, or if you awake at the end in the evening.

MEDICATION

The use of melatonin pills could appear to be a natural method to get sleepy, particularly when you're physically exhausted in the evening but not able to sleep. But, the majority of over-the-counter sleep aids contain three milligrams plus of melatonin, which is not enough. As per the Dr. Michael Breus (Board Certified Sleep Expert) during an appearance on The Dr. Oz Show, taking melatonin for self-medication could be harmful to your sleep habits and also your health. It may also trigger nightmares and should not be prescribed to children.

Melatonin is a hormonal hormone and may interfere with other hormones that are in your body If you're supplementing it and not making steps to fix the sleep issues you have.

Certain people use plain antihistamines, which cause drowsiness. They're considered safe when consumed "without any other components", i.e. there are no pain relievers or decongestants or expectorant. As they are only used for a couple of hours because tolerance quickly increases. They're not suggested as a permanent, long-term solution, but rather to "kick into gear" your return to an established routine of time, relaxation methods and reducing stress.

Be sure to read all the labelling and warnings that are printed on the medicine regardless of the length of time they last. It could affect your sleep (they might!) and you'll be in a loop of taking something that helps you sleep , but it's actually acting against you. Instead of taking the entire dosage that's listed on the label, consider taking a small portion to ensure you don't get an unpleasant hangover after taking the pills. It's best to be asleep the moment you take these medications and not out waiting for the effects to take effect'. Don't mix your medications. Consult your physician about possible interactions, or check it out on the internet before you do. You are responsible for your own health, and don't hand to anyone else your authority.

Make a list of your sleep issues so that you can let your doctor know. So that you don't forget any information. Let her know that you're worried about having some sort of sleep disorder. The most commonly reported sleep disorders include insomnia, heartburn, and narcolepsy (acid acid reflux). If you are suffering from any of thesedisorders, she will recommend the appropriate treatment.

In the short term natural sleep aids like valerian, tryptophan or soothing substances like passionflower or theanine may help you reset the body's rhythms.

About PETS

Yes my pets are as part of the family However, you shouldn't not be putting your sleep on your pet's security If they keep you awake at night or causing you to go out, or whining when you feed them.

It's not just me in the United States with regards to those who sleep together with animals. According to a survey conducted recently that found nearly half of dogs are sleeping in the beds of their owners. The survey revealed 60 percent of the small dog breed, forty percent of dogs of medium size, and three-quarters of the large breed rest with their owners.

The survey also revealed that sixty-two percent of cats rest with their adult caregivers, as well as another thirteen percent of cats are slept with by children.

Chapter 6: Techniques for Breaking Bad Habits That Trigger Sleep Issues

In the first chapter, two of them provided the essential information needed to comprehend sleep issues. The following chapters, however provide directions. They will guide you to the solution to insomnia. Learn more about HCCH cure and then you can get a good night's sleep.

What exactly does "HCCH" mean? It is the acronym for the four major aspects of your daily life that require more attention when you're trying to fight the sleep disorder that's common and these are:

Habits

Comfort

Calmness

Health

The remedy you'll to apply in your battle to combat insomnia, is easy as they come. And it is effective by targeting nearly every single possible source of the issue.

Tips to Break Your Bad Habits

The first hurdles you have to conquer is the habitual habits which hinder you from getting enough rest.

1. Recognize that you're suffering from an issue

If you're trying to change destructive habits, it is important to first acknowledge that they're actually harmful to you. Think about incidents that were traumatic and occurred because you're tired. Being a victim of a collision and being nearly cut while making food at home are just 2 "good" instances.

2. Make small, but specific goals

If you're looking at the screen with a wide-eyed look and awe-inspiring, affirm that it's the right time to make a change. Repeat your goals and the things you'd say repeatedly. Invoking "I'll never be watching TV until I'm asleep" and similar pledges will help make yourself believe that it's the time to change some aspects of your daily routine.

3. Stop Sleep Disorder Triggers

The act of uttering these words is not enough. Although you've made the conscious decision it is still up to your own mind to control. This is why you need to find methods to eliminate what causes the issue.

If, for instance, you frequently drift off into dreamland when watching TV, it is recommended to shift your TV into a more comfortable space. Another example is If you spend a lot of time working in your mattress (and then later fall to sleep) take everything that is related to work from your bedroom, and then begin to work elsewhere. In creating your personal habit-smashing strategies (and applying them) you'll be able to achieve two important things.

The first is all about cutting down on the urge. If there isn't a television within your room, then you'd be forced to rest properly. This is the same case for working productively while in mattress. If you're not being scolded from your notebook, you'll not have to write pages of reports until you fall asleep.

Apart from staying away from appealing (or or, in other words disturbing) objects, you'll be able to associate your bedroom solely with sleep. To be more specific, if you just see the area of your house as a spot for a peaceful sleep You won't see yourself engaged in any kind of activity instead of relaxing. It means you'll be able to sleep faster and longer.

4. Helping Others

What do you do if you've tried the methods you've developed to change your behavior and then relapsed to your old habits? If you're unable to alter the way you behave at your own pace then you should seek out help. It is possible to ask your loved ones to help you remember the things you should do, particularly when you're beginning to show indications of the possibility of a "relapse".

You can also have them create and follow their own lifestyle improvement plans to ensure that you don't feel at a loss in your fight against sleep disorders. Apart from receiving relatable support from your peers (and in turn) Your competitive side will also be rediscovered. It's not a good idea to see your friends ' improvements while you are the same.

Chapter 7: Sleep And Mental Health

Erratic Behavior patterns (mood swings) along with sleep is two sides one coin. One that can lead to the other in various circumstances. Insufficient sleep can cause irritability and short tempers mood swings, frustration and lack of attention at work or in other settings.

Research has proven that sleeping insufficiently is detrimental to mood. The research conducted by University of Pennsylvania. University of Pennsylvania found that those who displayed frequent indicators of stress, anger depression, sadness and fatigue were denied at least 4 to 5 hours of sleeping each night for a week. However, various levels of mental health demonstrate different degrees of harm that sleep has caused. Stress levels can raise alertness in the brain due to which the body is more anxious and stimulated. These people exhibit intense emotional reactions to stress. The mental stress acts as an inhibitor to stop sleep.

Sleep problems that are persistent are early indication that the person is headed for depression.

The people who suffer from insomnia are 20 percent more likely experience panic disorders that in extreme cases may develop into psychiatric disorders.

Do you worry about sleep?

Sleeplessness, also known as insomnia, is a chronic condition that makes it difficult to fall asleep, difficult to stay asleep , or both, in spite of a conducive environment to get a sufficient amount of sleep.

The person who suffers from this disorder typically wakes tired, unfocused and sluggish. It's not just a drain on your energy levels , but can may also affect your work and overall quality of life.

Different people require different amounts of sleep, according to their lifestyle and age.

The causes that can hinder the ability to sleep soundly include:

Utilization of stimulants, e.g. nicotine, cocaine, caffeine and excessive consumption of alcohol, certain drugs.

Mental health disorders, for instance bipolar disorders or depression clinically

Anxiety disorders like generalized anxiety disorder, or post-traumatic stress disorder

Disorders of the mind, such as schizophrenia, dementia.

The Side Effects of Insomnia:

The formation of weak brain cells: This can lead to memory loss which can result in a decrease in REM sleep, which promotes memory formation.

Poor Socialability : The repercussions of no sleep can cause an uneasy feeling of being deprived that makes us feel unfulfilling and socially awkward

Inattention and lack of concentration: leads to mental fatigue and concentration.

In turn, it prevents us from achieving our full potential.

Reduces Analytical Skills: Poor sleep may have a detrimental impact on our cognitive abilities that hinder the ability of our creative and critical thinking

Even though these damage can be very damaging to the body, you can take an elation as these damages are not irreparable. You can eliminate insomnia by making a few simple modifications to your day-to- daily routine, and by performing conscious mental exercises as a part of your routine.

Chapter 8: Mind, Body and Spirit: An Act of Reconnection

For many centuries practitioners of holistic healing were mostly ignored when they tried to explain the relationship between the body, mind and spirit operates. It's only been lately that research and science have grasped the concept. It has led to some important discoveries that have revealed connections to how patients deal with or recover from severe illnesses like cancer and heart disease. Researchers from the University of California at San Francisco (1) found that patients suffering from breast cancer who participated at weekly sessions of group therapy could live up to 2 times more than patients who didn't. In a different study, researchers from the University of California at Los Angeles discovered that patients undergoing cancer surgery for melanoma greatly benefitted from being educated about the reduction of anxiety levels, and coping techniques as well as weekly counseling. Patients who received these strategies had a 50 percent lower chance of recurrence, and 30 times less likely to be diagnosed with cancer and die.

Over the last 10 years, scientists from various universities around the world have examined the way that the body, mind and the spirit interact. There has been research that shows the benefits of prayer or even a simple meditation for people who don't adhere to any particular religion at the time of health crises. However, you don't need to be battling the risks of serious illnesses such as cancer to reap benefit from reconnecting. It is not necessary to be doing something "weird" or do anything you don't feel comfortable with. The goal is to restore a equilibrium, not to make an unbalanced one.

Before we go on Here are some crucial points to be aware of:

I'm not advocating one kind of religion over one. Actually, one doesn't need to adhere to a particular religion to have this connection. Even those who don't believe in religion or even atheists may be spiritually connected in a way that isn't tied to any god at all.

If you do not feel comfortable with any advice provided in this publication You are at ease to leave it out or modify it, or search for another option that works for you.

There isn't a single idea that works for everyone, so be aware of that also.

The first chapter of Chapter 1 discussed what happens following an evening of less than unrestful or disturbed sleep. We are tired or tired. We might forget little details. Sometimes, we do odd things such as putting keys to our car in the freezer, or place your butter into the washer as we're rushing to do the laundry. These are all annoying little items, but have you thought about why these events take place in the first instance?

We divide the body, the mind and the soul into three distinct parts, and assign them the same tasks. The brain is expected to assist us in remembering things and to be able to complete certain tasks, and also learn to accomplish other things. The brain is expected to prevent us from placing our keys to the car in the freezer, because it knows they don't belong there, yet here are our keys that are cold and icy every time.

Our body is expected to do physical activities throughout the day Naturally. We forget about the basic science classes in which we were taught that each movement is controlled by the brain through the vast nerve network. The body is treated as an instrument at times, but we forget that machines need to be recharged in some way to ensure they function properly.

From our souls we hope for the power to soothe us, provide us with nourishment and help our energy in times of intense stress. But, as we said we do not realize that we have to actively connect to that spirit in order in order for that connection to be present.

If your body is not well-rested, it could be injured. But, more importantly it is a sign that the mind hasn't had a the chance to recharge. If you're exhausted physically and mentally, there's no way to access your spiritual aspect. Find out how they're all linked to one another? A tense mood can hinder the sleep you need. Ailments or illnesses could prevent the sleeper from getting. Stress or anxiety can prevent your from staying asleep. By taking care of yourself, body, mind and spirit will restore your health, mental clarity, and your spiritual side back to normal.

Chapter 9: Treatments for Medical Conditions To Treat Sleepiness (Sleeping tablets/sleep aids)

Sleeping tablets , also known as sleep aids are medicines that aid people who suffer from insomnia sleep better. They are known as hypnotics. generally used to alleviate symptoms of insomnia in the short term and reduce the severe signs of insomnia, and also if other treatments are not able to be effective.

However, health professionals and doctors tend to be reluctant to recommend the use of sleeping pills or other sleep supplements to patients. While sleeping tablets may ease symptoms of insomnia, they do not solve the root of insomnia.

Sleep aids or sleeping tablets can't be effective for people suffering from long-term insomnia. The majority of doctors send these individuals to a sleep medicine specialist for other treatments.

If you're prescribed insomnia tablets your physician is likely to prescribe only the most minimal dose in the shortest amount of period, typically less than an entire week. If, however, you suffer from severe insomnia your physician is likely to suggest sleeping tablets 2 or 3 times per week instead of once a evening.

Sleep aids or sleeping tablets may also trigger side effects based on the kind dosage and the reactions of the person's body. They may cause an afternoon drowsiness, or even a feeling of hangover. Therefore, it's recommended to take sleeping tablets , or sleeping aids in the night prior to going to sleep.

In certain instances, particularly those who are older the feeling of a hangover will last into the following day. Therefore, it is recommended to take care in the event of driving on the next day or engaging in things that require active reaction.

Important Factors to Consider While taking sleep aids or sleeping Tablets or sleep Aids

Most of the time, people suffering from insomnia will are able to benefit from taking sleep aids or sleeping tablets to aid in falling to sleep, staying asleep through the night, or to improve the quality of their sleep. However there are a few aspects to be aware of when taking sleeping tablets or other sleep aids.

1. Sleep aids or sleeping tablets can be beneficial after you have tried non-medical or natural remedies, however insomnia remains and can disrupt your day-to-day activities.

2. A specific sleep aid may be recommended after your physician has determined the reason for your sleepiness. This means that you shouldn't just use a sleeping pill at your own will.

3. Sleep aids or sleeping tablets do not replace natural, healthy sleeping routines.

The most effective treatment for insomnia is to develop proper sleep habits. If you have a long-running insomnia you should remain on non-medicated treatments or a mixture of non-medical treatment as well as sleeping pills.

4. If you suffer from intermittent insomnia, sleeping tablets could aid. If your insomnia is something that happens for a short time, like jet lag, it's okay to take sleep aids. If your sleep issues persist for more than 3 days within a week, you must talk to your doctor and stop taking sleep aids.

5. Before taking sleep tablets or sleeping aids, consult your physician if you experience mental or physical health issues because of difficulty sleeping.

Certain sleeping tablets and sleep aids are available only on prescription. This is due to the fact that they could be addictive and could lead to more serious issues in the event that the form, dosage and dosage is not suitable for your specific insomnia issue.

Different types of sleep aids Tablets also known as sleep Aids

Benzodiazepines

These are drugs for insomnia which act as tranquilizers that can aid in promoting peace, sleep, and tranquility as well as reducing anxiety. Benzodiazepines are generally prescribed to those suffering from severe insomnia or stress because of insomnia.

The most frequent result of benzodiazepines can be sleepiness. Additionally, it could result in dependence or addiction which is the reason why doctors advise their use for the short-term effect.

Z Medicines

These medicines are short-acting which function in the same manner as benzodiazepines. They are regarded as the latest kind of medication for insomnia. They include zolpidemand zaleplon and zoplicone.

Zolpiden is a temporary medication for insomnia debilitating, and is generally recommended at the lowest dose for more than four weeks. A few of the most common adverse effects are headaches, fatigue, diarrhea sleep-related issues dizziness, nausea/vomiting and stomach discomforts. Some of the less frequently reported symptoms include double vision as well as a lack of concentration.

Zaleplon is a registered medicine for those who have trouble getting to sleep. It is typically given at the lowest dosage and is used for not more than two weeks. The side consequences of Zaleplon include insomnia as well as dysmenorrhea and painful periods for women, memory issues and paraesthesia such as pins and needles. The less frequent side effects of Zaleplon include a lack of balance and coordination and changes in perception of smell and hallucinations inattention or apathy difficulties in concentration, and dizziness.

ZOPICLONE is also an approved treatment for insomnia that is specifically designed for those who struggle with sleeping, awakening in the night, or suffering from suffering from debilitating insomnia. It is prescribed at the lowest dose and is taken for no longer than 4 weeks. The most common adverse effects of zopiclone are dry mouth, sleepiness and a metallic taste. The less frequent side effects of the medication include drowsiness, dizziness, headaches, vomiting and nausea.

Z medicines can also contribute to psychiatric reactions , including delusions, agitation aggression, anger as well as hallucinations, irritability, and sleep disturbances. If you experience any of these symptoms, stop taking these medications and talk to your physician whenever you can.

Antidepressants

Antidepressants are generally recommended to patients suffering from insomnia, especially in the event of a previous past history of depression. The most commonly used antidepressants prescribed to treat insomnia is the melatonin.

Melatonin is a melatonin-based medicine that has been shown to have a positive effect on effects of insomnia. Melatonin aids in controlling the cycle of sleep, referred to by the term "circadian rhythm" due to the fact the fact that it's a naturally occurring hormone.

Circadin is one of the more well-known medicine that is a mixture of melatonin. It is approved for the treatment of insomnia and available only with a prescription only for those older than 55. It is designed to treat insomnia for a brief period that is not longer than 3 weeks. If you suffer from kidney or liver disease it is not advised to use Circadin to treat insomnia.

A few of the adverse effects of Circadin include constipation, dizziness weight gain, anxiety, migraine, and stomach discomfort.

Alternative Medicines

There are a variety of alternative treatments for those who are having trouble sleeping or staying asleep through the night. However these drugs don't pass the same the same safety tests as other kinds of medicines. This means that their efficacy and potential side effects are not established or even understood.

Chapter 10: Sleep and the need for Sleep

Sleep disorders can be common but they don't need to affect you or your family's life. It is vital to know the importance of sleep and the best ways to manage sleep issues. Sleep can affect your body's function and mental health in a variety of ways. When you sleep your body could be unmoving, but your brain is alert throughout the day. Five phases to sleep.

The majority of adults spend half of their time sleeping in the second stage , or light sleep. Only 20 percent of their time in the REM stage, where the majority of dreams happen.

Infants however are able to spend the majority of their sleeping during their REM stage.

While you sleep your eyes will move slowly, and your muscles begin to relax.

In the initial phase of sleep, individuals can be easily woken.

In the next stage the eye stops moving and brain waves begin to slow. Stages 4 and 5 can be known as deep sleep, and it is very difficult to get someone awake.

In the REM stage breathing becomes more uneven and shallow. Eyes move in various directions, and muscles become temporarily frozen. The people who awake during REM are prone to bizarre dreams.

A complete sleep cycle could last up to 110 minutes.

When your sleep pattern gets disturbed, your body will not adhere to the normal cycle of sleep and immediately begins the REM sleep phase until your body is completely finished with this stage.

How long do you have to rest?

The amount of rest each person requires is contingent on various factors, including age. Children require 16 hours of sleep , while adults need at least seven to eight hours of sleep every evening.

Also, people require more sleep when they're not sleeping enough in the preceding days. If you are deprived of sleep, your body will need more time to sleep.

Although people may become accustomed to sleep-deprived circumstances, their performance may be affected. Research suggests that sleep-deprived drivers perform worse than those who are drunk when driving.

Benefits of sleeping

Sleep is essential to the survival of humans. A good amount of sleep is crucial to live the right balance of health. Sleeping better makes people feel healthier and able to take on more tasks during the day, and helps prevent under-eye circles. Here are a few of the most compelling reasons you should make sleeping one of your top priorities.

Enhances Memory

The mind is always active during sleep. You can enhance and build your skills while sleeping. If you're looking to master something new, you'll be able to do better when you are asleep.

Longer Life

In a study that was conducted recently, it was found that women between 50-79 years old who had under five hours of rest were more likely to die.

Helps to prevent inflammation

Inflammation is a cause of various diseases, including heart disease and arthritis. Patients who have less than six hours of rest are more likely to have elevated levels of inflammation-related proteins.

Enhances Creativity

In sleep the brain reorganizes itself and reorganizes memories, which can increase creativity. A study from Harvard University has shown that sleep enhances the emotional aspect of the brain which may boost creativity.

Sharpen Attention

Sleep deprivation can affect children in a different way. Although adults may feel tired but children tend to be active when they don't have enough sleep. This could cause them to be inattention and indecisive.

Healthy Weight

Anyone who is looking to shed weight should also think about extending the length of their sleep. Research shows that those who sleep more effectively lose weight. People who diet also experience more hunger when they don't get sufficient sleep. The reason behind this is that metabolism and sleep is controlled by the exact same region that controls the brain.

Lower Stress

Sleep can greatly reduce stress and also aid people in managing their blood pressure more effectively. It can also impact cholesterol levels and even helps reduce heart problems. Lack of sleep can cause depression. Find the right balance between functioning efficiently while getting sufficient sleep.

Chapter 11: The Basics Of Sleep Apnea and Snoring

Sleep apnea is a long-lasting condition that can be serious. your sleep is disturbed by breathing pauses, or when you feel your breathing is shallow during sleep. Breathing pauses can last from just a few seconds or minutes, and can occur at an average frequency of 30-35 times over an hour. If you stop breathing, the amount of oxygen reaching the brain is not as the normal. The brain reacts in this way by interrupting sleep, causing you to increase breathing. A loud gasping or choking sound can be heard accompanying this. Sometimes, this can cause the person to shift from a deep sleep and into a more relaxed sleep, or be awakened.

What are the different types of sleep apnea?

Obstructive sleep apnea is by far the most frequent kind. It is caused by the soft tissues in the back of your throat loosen when you sleep and can block the airway. In addition, allergies and other medical conditions that lead in nasal congestion and blockage can contribute to sleep apnea. If you suffer from this condition it is possible that you are not aware of the times you awake.

Central sleep apnea affects your central nervous system, and isn't as prevalent as sleep apnea with obstructive causes. It happens when the brain is unable to activate the muscles that regulate the breathing. Patients suffering from this condition do not have trouble sleeping and are generally conscious of their sleep being disturbed by apnea.

Complex sleep apnea can be described as the result of obstructive sleep apnea as well as central sleep apnea together.

Who is susceptible to sleep apnea?

Sleep apnea can be affecting males, females, young or old. There are specific risk factors that are associated with each.

There is a risk for Obstructive sleep apnea in the event that you:

older than 65

Male

Overweight

Smoker

Have you got a family member who suffers from sleep apnea?

Hispanic, Pacific Islander, or Black

Other elements could include the following physical characteristics:

Thick neck

Adenoids or tonsils that are larger (common for children)

The septum is deviated

The chin is receding

You could be at risk of central sleep apnea when you are:

Age 65 or over

who suffer from a severe medical issue (such as brain disease, heart disease suffering from a serious medical condition (such as the spinal cord or brainstem)

What are the symptoms and signs?

Sleep apnea can be the cause of an illness that is serious; therefore it is essential to see your physician. But, sleep apnea is not often recognized due to the fact that the symptoms most noticeable occur while you sleep. It is possible to seek the assistance of a partner in bed to track your sleeping patterns. You can also make recordings of audio or video of your the night. Sleep apnea can be a sign of sleep in addition to the following:

In the night, while asleep

breathless

breath stops

gasping for air or choked

awakenings, feeling confused

At daytime

Sore throat or dry mouth when you wake up

Morning headaches

Extremely sleepy

Sleep quality is not optimal.

Attention, concentration or memory

The mood swings

Recent weight gain

Do you think it's sleep apnea, or is it just the sound of snoring?

Snoring can be a sign of sleep apnea, however not everyone with sleep apnea also snore. Snoring does not necessarily mean that one suffers from sleep apnea. The main difference is being aware that the act of snoring is not necessarily interfere with sleep quality so daytime symptoms might not be evident.

What causes Snoring?

Snoring patterns can reveal the reason behind your snoring. If you can identify the reason for why you snore you'll be closer to determining the best treatment for your problem.

Snoring when the mouth is closed could indicate tongue problems

The fact that you are snoring while your mouth is opened could be due to the tissues that lie behind the throat.

Sleeping with your head on your back can be more mild and may be a sign of an adjustment in your posture and sleep routines, and lifestyle modifications

The snoring in all sleeping positions is more intense and could require more extensive control.

What are the best ways to treat sleep apnea , snoring and other sleep disorders?

The aim in treating sleep apnea is achieve the regularity of breathing patterns during sleep, and also to reduce symptoms like snoring or signs of poor quality sleep. Snoring and sleep apnea, both of which are obstruct can be addressed by making changes to your bedtime routine and life style, in addition to doing exercises for your throat. The use of clinical treatments is also looked at, and could include making use of a dental appliances as well as breathing devices, or even surgery. These medications are used only to treat sleepiness during the daytime that is associated with sleep apnea. It doesn't treat the apnea itself. If you suffer from central sleep apnea, treating the root medical issue, like heart or neuromuscular disorder is essential.

Chapter 12: A Science of Being Sleepy

Sleep is an integral aspect of our lives But do you know what causes it? A lot of sleep-related questions are being answered by science, however there are some aspects that remain a mystery. Let's look at the aspects you need to be aware of, particularly if getting to sleep is already an ongoing fight.

It is the Different Stages of Sleep

Neuroscientists, like those from Washington University in St. Louis classify sleep and the fall asleep and sleep itself into five phases: pre-sleep the transitional stage (or the stage one) and the non-REM stage (or Stage 2) the slow-wave sleep (or stages 3 and 4) and REM sleep. Each stage is explained briefly and in a non-technical manner as follows:

The pre-sleep stage. This is the stage where your"bedtime routine"transpires.

Particularly, it's the moment when you're just getting prepared for bed. It is the time to turn off the lights then settle down in your bed, and close your eyes.

When you are waiting for the time to fall asleep the brain goes through the transitional phase called"quiet wakefulness."In the same way it slowly shifts between thoughts of the external thoughts and your brain, and the former gradually becoming more dominant. These thoughts inside are self-reflection, or pure imagination or both.

At some point, usually after about 7 mins, it is when the brain shifts into The Transitional Sleep Stage.

This is known as the Transitional Sleep Stage. If you begin to dream without effort, you are probably in Stage 1, or the transitional stage of sleep. It's a fascinating state to be in since you may encounter what's called"hypnogogic hallucinations"in the shape of extraordinary but vivid thoughts and feelings. It is unclear what the duration of the sleep transition phase can last, but many speculate that it's between 5 to 10 minutes. If you are unable to sleep, you may then move into your sleep stage that is not REM. Sleep stage.

Non-REM Sleep Stage. This stage, often known as Stage 2 is the time when your body temperature decreases and your heart rate becomes lower. It also affects the brain's ability to see the external world. For example the music you be listening to in bed gradually diminishes in this stage.

The word REM is the abbreviation for"rapid eye movement,"which happens when you're in a dream. In this instance there is no the dreamland however. The stage will last about 20 minutes before moving on to the next one.

This is known as the Slow Wave Sleep Stage. If people talk about an extended, unrequited sleep it could be that they are referring to this stage. It was previously classified as Stages 3 and 4. It is also called"deep sleep" It is when the brain produces Delta Waves, also known as deep slower brain waves. It lasts about one-half hour, before transitioning into REM sleep.

This is known as the REM Sleep Stage. As you go deep into sleep your mind will reward your efforts by allowing you to go into the world of dreams. In this phase your muscles' voluntary ones are relaxed to the point of being inactive and you do not"act out"your fantasies. Your brain is on the other hand becomes more active. When you are in your first sleep cycle, this phase will last about 10 minutes. The more sleep cycles that you go through, the longer each REM sleep stage gets.

The transitional sleep stages as well as REM sleep last approximately one hour and thirty minutes. This is referred to in the context of one"sleep cycle."Throughout your sleep, you repeat the same cycle until you are able to wake up or are jolted out of it (as is the case with those who utilize the alarm clock).

How Do You Determine the Number of hours you'll need to sleep

The length of time you must sleep is determined by the amount of cycles your body and mind require. Be aware that yours is different from other.

Some, for instance, can manage with just three continuous sleeping periods (or four hours 30 minutes of rest) each night, but others require at minimum 5 hours of sleep (or more than 7 hours 30 mins).

To figure out the number of hours or cycles of sleep you require, keep track of the time at which you fell asleep during the previous night, and when you awoke the next day. Repeat this process for several nights (ideally over the course of a week). At the end of the test, you'll be able to gauge how many hours you must reserve for sleep each night. If you are unable to afford not to utilize an alarm clock at the beginning of your day then you could try this experiment during weekend when you can be able to get up without a need to be awake.

Once you have determined the number of hours you require then use that as a basis to develop your bedtime routine. For instance, if, for example, you observed that you typically get to sleep at about 11:00 p.m. and then get up around 6:30 a.m. This indicates that your body needs seven to 30 mins of rest or five sleep cycles.

If you need to get up by 5 a.m. to work, that means that you must make a count and then make your time for bed earlier. In this instance, it is on or before 9:00 p.m.

In addition aside from this, you must also consider the amount of time it takes you to sleep. If, for instance, you realize that you've fallen asleep after 20 minutes of getting to bed, you must be sure to allocate that amount of time for sleeping.

I hope that a majority of your concerns about sleep in your head are now answered and you are aware of how it works naturally. Make use of this knowledge to develop routines that allow you to get into the habit effortlessly. If you're not sure what to do, don't worry as the subsequent chapters of this book will guide you along the process.

Chapter 13: Devices And Surgery As Aids

For those who have chronic sleep apnea and the inability to begin an effective natural treatment There is a simpler and faster method of achieving a cure while you follow the slower , more long-lasting method. These tools will provide quick relief, but be sure to alter your lifestyle and follow the exercises mentioned in the final chapter.

As you have seen in the previous chapters there are three distinct types in sleep apnea. The devices that are mechanical here aren't all appropriate for all types of sleep apnea. If the issue is physical, that is, it's OSA The devices can provide the most effective relief. If the issue is more of a problem in the CNS, the devices won't offer much assistance and you'll require alternative solutions that are described in the following chapter.

CPAP to treat Sleep Apnea

The most popular treatment for moderate and serious cases OSA, CPAP or Continuous Positive Airflow Pressure makes application of a mask-like machine that provides a continuous flow of air. This allows breathing passages to be opened.

CPAP offers a compressor which is situated near the bed, and a hose which is strapped to a face mask that is worn on the forehead. This mask has an airtight seal which is then able to transfer air from the compressor to the nose at a pressure. The pressurized air is then able to keep the nasal passages open. The higher pressure increases the diffusion of oxygen through these passages through increasing the pulse oxygen levels. The positive pressure that is created in the airways allows breathing to flow smoothly and sleep to remain uninterrupted. This is clearly a solution to OSA as opposed to CSA.

It is important to note that CPAP isn't the most comfortable to wear, and many patients experience it as an issue at night.

Tips to Adjust to the CPAP Unit

Before you do that, make sure the mask is in good fit. If the mask is comfortable and comfortable, it's much easier to wear all night. When the face mask fits too tightly, it could feel uncomfortable. It can take time to determine the proper fitting.

In the second, you should give yourself time to adjust to the discomfort. It will be apparent that the discomfort you feel is well worth the extra sleep. There is no need to force yourself into using the mask. It is perfectly normal to be uncomfortable having the mask on to sleep. It is best to wear it for short durations during the entire day.

Third, personalize the device to your preferences. The components of the CPAP device, such as the mask, straps and tubing can be adjusted to ensure you get the perfect fit. Additionally, there are soft pads. These pads are helpful in reducing irritation to the skin as consequence of wear and tear. There are also nasal pillows as well as chinstraps that can help reduce the chance of irritation to your throat.

Fourth, apply it using an humidifier. A specific moisturizer can be applied prior to going to go to bed. Actually, the most recent models of CPAP have been fitted with an integrated humidifier.

Other devices for breathing recommended to help sleep Apnea

Sleep experts may also suggest different breathing devices. This could comprise Bilevel Positive Airway Pressure (BPAP) and Adaptive ASV. (ASV).

BPAP (or Bilevel Positive Airway Pressure

This is an alternative in place of CPAP particularly for patients who have difficulty to get used on it. CPAP unit.

It is BPAP was designed in order to regulate the pressure of the air as the patient lies down. If the patient breathes the device, it provides greater pressure. When it is the case that you (the patient) exhale the device is able to adjust and reduces the air pressure. The devices are BPAP devices designed to aid the patient to breathe once more after the device detects that the patient hasn't breathed for a few minutes.

The BPAP is a viable option for people suffering from CSA. Since when you suffer from CSA the brain stops telling that breathing muscles do their job the required actions, the BPAP continues to push in air to the lungs at the appropriate pressure. It's like a ventilating device which detects whether that patient's breathing or not, and then supplies air in order to compensate.

ASV, also known as Adaptive Servo-Ventilation

For those suffering from sleep apnea that is central or obstructive, ASV devices can monitor and record data about the patient's breathing patterns. It provides airflow pressure that is designed to stop breathing pauses. This can be one of the most dangerous symptoms of the condition.

Oral Appliances to help sleep Apnea

Dental devices are dental appliances which are used in place in place of CPAP or other medical devices. These devices are more static since they are placed in your mouth patient and stay there for a while. This is similar to braces that alter the shape of the teeth's profile. They're not moving, but they are always applying pressure to alter the shape of the teeth.

For OSA the devices are made to ensure that the throat stays open since the throat is prone to relax. A relaxed throat can lead to the condition known as apnea. There are a variety of designs of oral appliances. Certain are designed to move your jaw inwards. This is a mechanism that can assist in opening the throat. While oral appliances are efficient, they might not be as efficient as CPAP devices.

The majority of the devices made out of acrylic. They fit in the mouth, similar to the mouthguards that many athletes wear. There are additional devices that can be placed in the chin or head. One of the more commonly used devices for dentistry currently are the tongue retaining device and the mandibular-repositioning device.

The primary purpose of these devices is to pull the tongue and lower jaw forward, keeping the air passages open during sleep. They help by enhancing the tone of the tongue's muscles and repositioning the tongue the lower jaw and uvula, and soft palate.

Oral appliances are merely more comfortable than heavier and bulkier devices like CPAP. It takes much time to adjust to the devices in comparison to CPAP which can take a few months to adjust. A couple of weeks to become accustomed to it is enough. Since these dental devices are small they're also easy to carry around.

Commonly prescribed for mild to moderate sleep apnea cases, dental devices can cause adverse effects, including nausea, soreness, accumulation and mouth smell.

Surgery for Sleep Apnea

Surgery is generally considered the last option. Surgery should be considered only after having exhausted all other options for treatment. Surgery can be used to expand the airway's size that can decrease the frequency of sleep apnea-related episodes.

Here are some steps:

Shrinking

If a patient has an excessively enlarged airways the procedure of shrinking can be carried out. Somnoplasty for instance, utilizes radio frequency ablation for shrinking the palate soft, turbinates and uvula of the nose, the base of the tongue, and the Uvula.

Stiffening

Stiffening procedures are typically performed via implants. It is a possibility for those suffering from sleep apnea who have a soft palates that can disrupt the airway. The implants are generally composed of plastic, and are generally inserted in the rear of the mouth, or inside the mouth's soft palate.

Repositioning and removal

Other procedures involve the elimination of tonsils, adenoids and any extra tissue found within the nose or behind the throat. Repositioning procedures are also done. For instance, the jaw could be moved or rebuilt to create more space for the airway in the upper.

Before you decide to undergo surgery, make sure that you are fully informed about the procedure. Make note of what you can anticipate. Be aware that surgery is usually accompanied by some risks as well as complications. There is always the possibility of an infection. However, if you select your surgeon with care and maintain a healthy lifestyle prior to and following the surgery, you will significantly reduce your risk.

Chapter 14: The Health Benefits of Sleep That You Do Not Know About

Okay, we are all aware of what sleep is however do we understand what happens during the realm of nodding? Instead of being a state of consciousness, our bodies undergo many different processes that allow us to function efficiently as human beings throughout the rest of our lives.

Sleeping is a time of rest that permits the body to cleanse and undergo vital repair. Insufficient sleep can result in unhealthy health for many of us. According to health experts that those who sleep for five hours or less have a lower life expectancy than those who are able to sleep for more than six hours every night. We can conclude that sleep plays a crucial part to play in our mental and physical health.

Even though we're asleep (mostly) or in a state of dormancy, the brain is very active throughout our sleep, but of course, not as much as when we are awake, but the brain activity remains about 60% that we normally activity.

The research has revealed that the brain goes through various cycles, with different levels of brain waves which transmit signals to different areas of our bodies while we sleeping. The two primary phases include Non rapidly moving the eye (NREM) along with rapid eye movements (REM). There are five phases of sleep that happen during NREM along with REM.

When we are in NREM which is about 70% of evening sleep, we go through four phases of sleep. The first phase is basically sleeping, which includes our going to bed and drifting off to a restful sleep as we get to sleep.

The second phase is sleeping properly the heart rate becomes normal as our temperature falls. Also, we become less aware of the surrounding environment because we enter an unconscious state.

This brings us to step 3 , 4 and 5 of our sleep cycle. In this stage, we are asleep to the fullest extent of the night. Our blood pressure is lower as well as our respiration slows down. It is the single most critical aspect of sleep because most of the recuperative process is carried out by the body and brain. The muscles relax which results in increased blood flow to these areas, causing the repair of damaged tissues. In this stage, your energy levels are getting restored so that we can take on the next day's challenges. The hormones are also released, particularly if we are still in our formative years, and these hormones promote growth in our bodies.

The second and final stage is referred to as REM. While the eyes are closed, the eyes are flitting in fast movements. The the brain's activity levels are at their peak at this point and this is the time when we are most likely to sleep. There are also periods of breathing that are irregular and heart rate is unpredictable too. In this case, however, our muscles become paralyzed, preventing the movement of muscles.

The 5 phases mentioned above could be divided into three phases of sleep , which are described below.

Energy Conservation, Restoration, and Brain Plasticity

Sleep, first and foremost, assists your body in replenishing itself through a multi-faceted procedure of energy preservation. Harvard University researchers have highlighted three primary functions of sleep which include the conservation of energy, body rejuvenation and brain plasticity. The concepts might sound complex and difficult to comprehend in a glance, however you've surely observed their impact on your health. When you sleep, your energy needs and expenditure decreases. This is a natural process in animals and humans. While we are asleep our metabolism slows down and the body will save energy.

While it could appear to be one process, it is actually a different result of sleeping. Our body expends energy and is 'used up in the routine things we do when we're awake. It's all about energy and the structure of cells here. If you're looking to get an understanding of the rejuvenating effects of sleep, consider the force of your muscles when you're exhausted and then compare it to the tone you feel after a great night's sleep. In the same way, you can observe the rejuvenating effects of sleeping for your face. Cell rejuvenation is among of the primary results of a restful night and it happens on numerous levels in your mind and body.

It's not just the appearance on your face that could be enhanced by good sleep as well as your overall health. Did you realize that animals are susceptible to die if they're not getting enough sleep for long periods of period of time? This is explained by the connection between sleep and immunity function. In addition the hormonal balance of your body is maintained during your sleeping. Your sleep is the base for a variety of vital processes within your body. For instance, protein synthesis occurs during our sleep.

Another important effect of sleep that Harvard researchers studied was brain plasticity. This phenomenon is much more advanced and is related to the fact that sleep enhances the structure and structure of brain functions in subtle ways. The primary factor contributing to this is a stage called REM. The brain in our dreams is able to participate in complex actions that simulate real-life scenarios and actions. This is why REM can provide a higher amount of creativity and flexibility. Our ability to dream as well as the activities that take place within our minds as we are asleep enhances our brain's general capacity for plasticity and ability to complete different kinds of tasks throughout the daytime. Be aware that your brain doesn't go into a state of total inactivity while we sleep! It is still acting on its own and play various movies in our minds. This kind of numb however, quite intricate action that follows a logic of its own is believed to boost our brain's capability of focusing on a variety of kinds of tasks throughout the daytime. It's like if your brain did some silent practice while you slept!

Hormonal Activity Aside from the health benefits of sleeping There are many ways that the quality and length of your rest can aid you in living better and longer. The most significant factor can be the production and stimulation of different hormones within the body when you sleep. Like, for instance, well recognized and vital growth hormone was created to aid the body's development while we sleep. This is the reason why children sleep lots and the growth of their bodies is related to this process within the body.

But, the growth hormone is also beneficial for adults. The better your sleep, the better you'll avoid the atrophication of muscles and the healthier you can keep your tissues and cells. This isn't always immediately apparent but it is definitely there. It's difficult to determine whether the muscles in your body are strong and/or weak after you've slept for 8 hours. However, you must take note of the long-term benefits of a healthy sleep. If you are able to improve your sleep routinely and enjoy all the benefits The condition of your tissues will definitely improve.

It is a scientifically-proven result that can be attributed in part to the release different hormones in the sleep. In the same way, the hormones for sex increase in the night, which can lead to an increase in sexual desire and energy. In the case of men, this could play a significant role on sexual problems. Many people have realized that lack of sleep could cause erectile dysfunction, and decrease sexual desire. Sleeping well can regulate your sex hormones , and in turn, your overall sexual life.

Memory and Learning

The most intriguing and extensive benefits of a good sleep is the ability to remember and learn. We are all aware that we've performed better on tests or in presentations after a few hours of sleep. But, a regular sleep routine can boost the general quality of your memory as well as ability to learn. The benefits may not be apparent at first but they're still powerful. Studies show that sleep affects memory processing and how we process and remember events or information.

This is crucial from a variety of aspects: sleep helps you to'store' facts you must be able to recall, while also organizing information in a way you can find it and utilize it whenever you need. In addition sleeping well can improve your memory in an emotional way: your overall mood, mood as well as your comprehension and perception what you are experiencing can depend on the quality of sleep you're getting.

If you're exhausted and drained, your brain may drift around in circles and cause you to recall predominantly negative incidents, which puts you in a negative mood. It is the reason a restful night is recommended for the capacity to assess things objectively, and to ensure that your memory isn't influenced by an excessive bias of emotion. Sleep plays a major part in the storing/consolidation stage of our memory processes. You gather facts and remove them from your memory to use them while you're awake. But, the storage of data and organization has been proven to be improved by quality sleep. That's what researchers have told us. For performance and learning the immediate as well as long-term routines are involved If you have enough sleep, you will perform better at your studies as well as at work.

Your concentration, your attention power, your vigilance and your capacity to work using data are all improved when you've had a good night's sleep. However , getting enough rest regularly can affect our cognitive abilities and capacity to complete tasks and to acquire new information. The brain is relaxed and open to new knowledge that we are able to store without conscious thought in a more organized way. All we need to do is ensure we are aware of what good sleep is, and then we will be able to enhance the memory of our brain and improve our learning capabilities!

Sharp Focus and Rapid decision-making

Sleeping better will aid you in any circumstance that demands sharp focus and quick decision-making e.g. driving, sports, contests, exams etc. Researchers have found that lack of sleep could affect our brain in a manner similar to drinking alcohol. So any scenario which requires concentration and speed can be positively affected by a good night's sleep, from contests to business meetings and job interview. And lastly, but certainly not least the ability to think more clearly is enhanced by better speaking ability when you have peaceful sleep. Sleeping well people are more articulate and efficient. Consider this aspect of your nightlife as you consider whether that you can perform better in performance or presentation.

Skin Health

One of the greatest advantages of sleep is its effects on the health of your skin. Sleeping helps to replenish the tissues of your body and helps reduce dark circles and wrinkles. It can soothe dry skin, and can aid in the treatment of your skin by itself - in essence, many unwelcome skin issues, including sunburn, irritation and pimples may be less noticeable when you have a restful and restful sleep. The skin can learn to recycle itself' in the sleep. Naturally, you must use regular methods of skincare. Remember how important sleep is!

Emotional Control and Stress Relief

Sleeping well helps people manage stress better. They are able to see things clearly and can remain at peace even when faced with stressful situations. A better night's sleep can help you to avoid emotions like anger, anxiety or even indignation. This will positively impact your relationships as well as your efficiency at work. A sound sleep also balances your mood and assists you to overcome depression or anxiety attacks. Also, sleep can be described as an emotion regulator which operates independently of your conscious process. Naturally, if you are experiencing a tough moment, it is recommended to seek help from a professional or look for other options to treat your problem. But, remember that a better night's sleep can assist you in getting rid of anger or negative feelings.

All-Soothing for Various Types Of illness

Sleeping in doesn't just relieve your mind from stress, but it also eases migraines by giving your brain and body to recover. It's been proven that those who don't have enough sleep experience more headaches than others. While this is something to take with a pinch or two of salt. Some studies indicate that good sleep can assist you deal problems with health issues like diabetes or heart issues. It is believed that a restful night may lower the blood pressure. This reduces the chance of a heart attacks. This is why people with heart issues must ensure they are sleeping well and for long enough. Between 8 and 9 hours of sleep each night are the foundation of a heart that is healthy. It is also believed that sleep helps reduce cholesterol levels, not just heart pressure and is a proven way to avoid or prevent heart disease.

A Instrument in Cancer Prevention

The result of good sleeping could be keeping cancer-related risk at bay, no matter how unbelievable as it might sound initially. If the cancer virus is such a ferocious adversary, how can be it fought off with such a simple and readily available weapon? If you are already sick sleeping alone won't aid in the treatment. But, a schedule of a perfect night's sleep is believed to aid individuals in this regard. When you sleep (especially those who sleep in total dark) your levels of the hormone melatonin within your body rise and block the growth of cancerous cells in the long-term. So a regular, good sleep can assist in avoiding cancer, specifically breast and colon cancer.

Hormone Activation

As you've already observed numerous hormones are able to find the perfect place to go within your sleeping. It sounds quite easy, doesn't it? The hormones in your body are more active when you are doing nothing. That's why it is possible to lose weight or keep fit by sleeping. If you're wondering whether this is a joke, it's not. Research has shown that those who are able to sleep for long and well enough remain slim, as sleep enhances levels of leptin inside the body.

Are you aware of the number of individuals (especially women) are struggling to bring this hormone up to a higher level and shed weight? Leptin is the hormone responsible for the regulation of appetite, and is typically associated with a successful method of losing weight which can last for a long time. Therefore, bringing your sleeping routines up to a high standard is vital in order to remain healthy and fit with minimal effort! Research suggests that people who do not get more than 7 hours of sleep each night could suffer from lower levels of leptin and consequently suffer from unwelcome weight-related issues.

Another hormone released in the course of sleep is cortisol. If cortisol levels aren't high your skin is susceptible to fine lines, wrinkles and a lack of tone. Cortisol aids your body in breaking down collagen proteins that play a role in the aging processes that affect your skin. Along along with growth hormone cortisol and collagen are both essential to maintaining healthy skin. So, a good night's sleep and more will help keep your skin healthy through an increase in the right hormones within your body.

As you will observe, there are a myriad of reasons to try the best you can to get better rest. Not only will your overall health improve with the enhancement of your immune processes and body rejuvenation as well, but you also can quickly achieve a positive psychological state through a good night's sleep.

In simpler terms sleeping better can aid in making you more relaxed and less susceptible to illness or stress by triggering a myriad of natural processes that your body defends, maintains or heals itself. From improved concentration and memory to a healthier and younger body, the advantages that this chapter highlighted will be worth the effort to alter your sleeping habits to your benefit.

What should you do? Do you have a lot of questions? Are other aspects of your life affected as well? There are solutions to these questions in the following chapter, which will inform you about the most effective methods for improving your sleep and provide you with some suggestions and tricks that to use if you are looking to improve your sleep.

Chapter 15: Different Types Of Sleep And Sleep Cycles

You may be thinking "what is a silly book title, most likely you're asleep, or aren't". It's not true. There have been numerous studies conducted on the way that humans sleep and it's been discovered to be a much more complicated science than it appears initially. There is no sense when we shut our eyes and go to bed and fall asleep, we enter deep sleep, instead it has been discovered that we go through a sequence of rhythms of sleep, along with associated motions, all of that are crucial to waking up the next day feeling refreshed or not. It is essential to gain at least some understanding of these in case you're having trouble with sleeping - whether it is a problem getting into bed at all or waking up in the middle of the night or even other issues. In the remaining chapter , we will explore the different stages and patterns of sleep.

Circadian Rhythm - Our Body Clock

To understand the way we sleep, how we are exhausted, etc. we must understand the reasons behind why we are tired at certain periods of time. All living things have an internal unconscious, but usually conscious, response to external events and their environment. In a simplest sense, this implies that the changes occur in direct relation to the day's rhythms generally when it is bright and dark. Of course, this is subject to change. Find out why it is that the most activity in the world's natural ecosystem occurs at night. Birds chirp when the sun is rising (or somehow, they are aware that they are getting closer) and then they chirp when the sun sets and they go back to rest. Humans, naturally are part of the natural world , too and, in general, adhere to the natural patterns that are associated with the sun and daylight , however, for a large portion of humanity it is possible to change the length for which it is at night and how bright.

For humans, then these vital rhythms occur over a 24- hour period, and this more general phenomenon is referred to by The Circadian Clock. In reality, light and darkness are the primary factors that determine our state of mind when we're awake, and exhausted, although there are other factors that influence our mood. You may feel more exhausted after working hard, and other times, but the underlying factor behind this is the natural sleep cycle that is influenced by our surroundings, which impacts everyone. We've spoken a bit about shift working before and in the end, these ways of working could interfere with the natural rhythms of our bodies, and it is this that could cause shift work to be particularly harmful - in the meantime, you may be unable to sleep at night, in contrast to the natural rhythms. It is crucial to do your best to ensure that there aren't excessively unnatural influences on your body's clock and we'll discuss this in a bit later.

Sleep phases

Once you have an understanding of yourself, your insomnia, your sleeping patterns and the basic physics that is the Circadian Clock, we can begin to explore the various phases of sleep. This will bring us back to our previous remarks about the fact that sleep isn't identical - if you consider it, this could be the reason the reason why, for instance you might have stayed sleeping all night and still be tired when you wake up and exhausted. It's possible that you didn't get sufficient amount of sleep that you require to be fully rested. Let's look at the various kinds of sleep, and then try to discern what's taking place before you go to bed.

When you get to sleep, you be in an interval of non-rapid eye movements (NREM) sleeping. Research has shown that this sleep phase is divided into three distinct stages in which each one causes you to fall deeper sleep, meaning it becomes more difficult to wake up (and it can be confusing if you wake awake during this stage). Typically, the third and final stage of sleep that you'll enter will be the one called fast eye movements sleep (or REM). This is usually the phase of sleep that most people are most familiar with and at this point, you'll have come out of a deep sleep and could be nearing being awake. At this point, that you'll realize that you're in a dream. As per the Sleep Council, each of these four stages takes about 90 minutes, and a restful night can be expected to have the cycle of five or six that must include all stages in need to go through in order to get well refreshed. If you've experienced a shaky night's sleep or don't go to bed in a long enough time and you don't feel rested . This is why it is crucial to ensure you attain the necessary hours of sleep that you require and we'll discuss the next.

How much sleep do I need?

The whole discussion of the stages, phases, and cycles of sleep make it seem as if there's plenty going on when we are asleep! There are times when there is however, the main aspect is to ensure that you give yourself enough time to get the proper amount of time to sleep that are most suitable for your. The amount of sleep you require will be contingent on a range of variables among them the most crucial aspects to consider is the age you are. These are the recommended amount of rest.

For newborn babies, from three months to three months approximately 14 to 17 hours is the recommended amount of time, although it is possible that slightly higher or lower may be appropriate . Typically during the early days , a baby will awake and fall asleep in short bursts in order to adjust to the Circadian Clock that we have discussed earlier. As the baby grows older, typically between four and 11 months, the need for sleep decreases by a bit, but it is still between 12 and 15 hours, with a certain latitude over and below this number.

As children learn how to move and walk about between the ages between one and two then the minimum requirement decreases again between 11 or fourteen hours. It is important to note that these are only minor and gradual shifts. At the point that the child is around just one or two years old they'll probably be taking one or two nap times during the day and the longer sleep at night - however, this can differ from child to child. From the age of pre-school, which is three to five, the typical hours range from 10-13 hours. The changes are likely to be less obvious between the years of between six and 13, with timeframe for the core hours likely to be in the range of nine to eleven hours however, again with an option to either increase or decrease. Teenagers will need less sleep however you could discover that this is not the case, or the patterns of sleep are different and often due to hormonal issues. Adults of all ages generally require at minimum seven hours of sleep and as long as nine hours. Some might require more, others a little less. Once you reach the age of 65 one can expect that a person will still need more than seven hours of rest but could be able get a bit less than the younger adults.

It's only an outline and what works for an individual of a certain time will not necessarily work for the other. This is why it's crucial to know your personal needs and take the necessary steps to reach your sleep goals.

Chapter 16: The diagnosis of sleep Apnea

The diagnosis of the problem can be challenging, since the majority of people think that it is an unrelated snoring issue. If you're among those with the symptoms listed above, you must attempt to get them evaluated. Here are some of the most common ways to determine Sleep Apnea.

Polysomnogram

A polysomnogram (PSG) is a sleep test that is used for detection of Sleep Apnea. It is a method of the monitoring of brain activity, heartbeats eye movements, and levels of blood pressure in the patients. The levels of oxygen of your blood may be determined using this method. The chest movements of the patient will indicate whether he's breathing normally or not. If it's observed that the patient needs additional effort to breathe normally this could indicate a sign or a symptom of

Sleep Apnea. A lot of times, doctors conduct the "split-night" study, in which the CPAP machine is utilized during the second part of the study to determine.

Portable Monitors

A portable monitor is handy to determine if you suffer from Sleep Apnea or not. The monitor is extremely popular because of its easy operation and small size. It helps document similar data to that offered by the PSG method, without having to travel to an office to have the test performed. The monitor, which is portable and home-based, will detect the following aspects:

A) Levels of oxygen present in blood

B) Rate of heartbeat

c)Airflow is a movement of air across the nose when taking a breath

d)Easy or challenging chest moves

Sleep Studies

Sleep studies are an exhaustive analysis of a patient's sleeping patterns. It determines whether the patient has a good night's sleep or if it is disrupted by the patient having to wake up often. By studying this it becomes much more clear what is the causes of the patient's erratic sleep patterns. Doctors also need to examine how severe the disorder is before prescribing the right dosage of treatment.

Physical Exam

Physical examinations are essential to determine Sleep Apnea problems in children as they exhibit obvious physical symptoms of the condition. Tonsils that are large can be easily detected through a physical examination which allows the doctor to examine the nose, mouth and tonsils in the patients.

Many times you might suspect you suffer from insomnia, but it may turn into sleep apnea. You could be confused by the symptoms of other illnesses or conditions and end up identifying it as a typical issue.

Let's create an inventory of the most crucial questions you could consider to find out the precise cause of your sleeping in a slumber or having a lot of sleep.

Quiz to determine if you suffer from Sleep Apnea

1.) Do you snore every day or at least 3 times during the week?

A) Yes

B) No

2.) Do you snore disturb the sleep of others?

A) Yes

B) No

3)Are you suffering from at least three of the mentioned sleep apnea signs?

A) Yes

B) No

4.) Do you have an unusual habit of sleeping during the daytime?

A) Yes

b)No

5) Does your collar's size significantly larger than the other collars?

A) Yes

B) No

These questions can assist you in determining whether your snoring issues are caused by Sleep Apnea. If you're able to answer yes more frequently than otherwise, then there's an excellent chance that you suffer with Sleep Apnea and need to seek out a physician immediately.

Chapter 17: The Way to Dream Lucid Dreams Fundamental Facts

It is normal to dream that happens when you are able to sleep regardless of whether it's deep or shallow. It is likely that you have been aware of this phenomenon they refer to as LD or Lucid dreams. Are you fascinated by it? There's a high possibility that all you've got to this point are theories regarding LD. Many believe it's real controlled and imagining. Some claim that this is the way people achieve OBE which is also known as Out of Body Experience. Do you agree? What do you think of dreamlike dreams?

Let's take a look at the fundamental details on it during this article. To simplify lucid dreams are all about dreaming and being aware of it. Are you still confused? For a more straightforward explanation the person suffering from LD is asleep , however they are aware that the events being experienced or heard appear to be part of the dream. Have you ever had a dream that you were flying, and later discovered that this is actually true and that you'll never be in danger of falling? The realization that you recognized it as a possibility in your head and were having fun while doing it indicates that you were lucidly dreaming.

A specialist in this area, Frederick Van Eeden, described lucid dreams to be "mental Clarity". When one is experiencing dream lucid, every detail is recalled with an astonishing level of clarity and precision. Typically, the state of clarity is reached in the mid-point of the dream. It happens when someone is able to see that what's that is happening can't be possible in normal conditions. It could occur even when there are no clues. Sleep researchers have discovered about 10% of the dreams can be experienced can occur after returning to REM sleep after having been suddenly awakened.

Two levels are of lucidity you can attain when you dream. They are:

The High-Level Lucidity (HLL) The state of being in which there is an absolute consciousness that everything happening is a part of the dream you are living. It is an understanding that physical harm can be averted as well as that, at any point you'll awake.

The Low-Level Lucidity (LLL) A kind of lucidity happens when you're aware only to a certain extent that you're dreaming. In this case, you don't realize that you are able to change the circumstances that are present or that there's no danger of physical harm by what you're doing.

Then, why do we talk about lucid dreams? Are there any advantages can be derived from this entire process? The answer is yes. There are numerous reasons that lead us to be attentive to getting clear dreams. Take a look at the following:

Allows for safe adventures and enjoyable adventures: LD enables an individual to live out their fantasies within a safe and secure setting. For instance, flying is among the most frequently-dreamed of fantasies for numerous people.

helps in overcoming nightmares: Realizing that the elements you fear in a dream could actually assist a person to overcome nightmares. Lucid dreams are utilized by sleep therapists to assist individuals face their fears.

Helps prepare individuals for real-life situations: This is referred to rehearsal. The scenario may be as realistic as we've ever imagined that we could make use of it to simulate anticipated or feared situations. Public speaking, sports performance as well as interviews can be practiced through LD.

Increases brain's creativity and problem-solving abilities: LI (Language International) researchers have discovered that students of language who are who are exposed to LD are more responsive to word-related connections. Lucid dreamers are also observed in a different field of research as more daring in coming up with work of art.

Improves physical health: Lucid dreams may help in healing the body. The healing dreams of lucid dreaming can stimulate the body to concentrate more on healing injuries and the practice of physical activities temporarily lost because of injuries, or simply help an injured person have optimism about his situation.

It is a source of transcendental experience It assists an individual to explore the spiritual side of life. The aim of seeking the purpose of life could begin in dreams that are lucid.

Lucid dreaming isn't just an uneasy topic for many but it also offers fascinating benefits as we have seen in the previous paragraphs. How can you get lucid dreams with purpose? Read the next chapter to find out more about it!

Chapter 18: Risk factors and causes of sleep Apnea

Sleep apnea is a condition that can affect anyone however there are certain categories of people at risk of developing this particular condition. Here's a list factors that can cause the person for developing sleep apnea

* Sleep apnea due to gender is more prevalent in males due to the fact that they have larger necks as compared to women. Men are also more weighed than women. Women however are susceptible to sleep apnea following menopausal changes since they tend to gain weight and grow in the size of their necks at this point.

* Age-related - the condition is more prevalent among people between 40 and 60 years old, and that's when the symptoms are most severe. Sleep apnea, however, can be a concern for anyone from all ages.

* Race - within the United States, this condition is more prevalent among African-Americans. Pacific Islanders and Mexicans are different groups that are at a higher risk of the development of sleep apnea.

* Obesity-related - overweight people tend to be more predisposed to develop the condition.

Smokers who smoke two packs or more in a day are more at risk of developing sleep apnea. Smokers are 40% more likely to suffer from this disorder when compared with non-smokers.

*Hereditary - the presence of sleep apnea among family members is an additional risk factor for developing this disorder.

* Alcohol Drinkers sleep apnea can be closely linked with alcohol and people suffering from sleep apnea should be advised not to consume alcohol before going to bed.

• Medical conditions – some medical conditions are the main cause of sleep apnea. Here are a few medical conditions that can cause sleep apnea

Obesity - it is connected with sleep apnea, snoring and sleep disturbances. But, it hasn't yet been determined if there's a real connection between the two conditions or if it's due to the weight problems that plague many diabetics.

It is also known as Gastro Esophageal Reflux Disease (GERD) This is a condition in which the acid is flowing throughout esophagus. This is one of the causes of sleep apnea because the back up of stomach acid in the esophagus triggers spasms in the larynx which creates a blockage in the airway to the lungs , creating apnea.

O Polycystic Ovary Syndrome - this has been identified as an important risk factor that contribute to sleep apnea because women who suffer from PCOS suffer from diabetes, and it is linked to sleep apnea.

* Large Neck - the neck of a person is 17 inches or greater in males , and 16 inches or more for females, is an indicator of sleep apnea.

Once you have a better understanding of the risks of sleep apnea, it is possible to investigate the root cause. Sleep apnea can be caused by any one or more of these:

* Structural Abnormalities is one of the major causes of sleep apnea that is obstructive. These abnormalities are:

O Micrognathia - chin with a small size

A narrow upper jaw

The Retrognathia, lower jaw that juts

o Large tongue

• Tonils that have been enlarged

* The characteristics that are characteristic of Soft Palate - the abnormalities in the structure of the palate in the rear part of the throat and mouth could be the cause of sleep apnea. The most likely cause is

the soft palate is more rigid and/or larger. The reason could come due the soft palate or throat wall around it are prone to collapse.

* Obstructions that are either total or partial in the airway because of the following:

Larger tonsils or a tongues that could cause obstruction if it is bigger than the the windpipe's opening

O Fat tissues that could make the wall of the windpipe which can narrow it.

The shape of the head and neck size could result in a narrowed passage between the throat and mouth.

*The Aging Process - this may result in your brain sending wrong signals, which could cause narrowing or collapse of the airway, thereby creating airway obstruction.

* Muscle weakness - this could cause sleep apnea when muscles relax and cause obstructions to the airway.

Sleep apnea causes in children are as these:

Anomalies in skull or facial structures are a cause of sleep apnea for the population of younger age. This includes the brachycephaly.

Tonils that are too large or Adenoids are also a reason for sleep apnea in kids. Removal of both can open the airway and resolve sleep apnea.

* Diseases that affect the neuromuscular system which affects the muscles that are found within our airways.

These are just a few of the factors that contribute to being a victim of sleep apnea. If you're prone to these issues and notice signs of sleep apnea arising in your life, it could be time to seek assistance before it dramatically impacts your health.

Chapter 19: The Symptoms of Sleep Apnea

How do you tell if you suffer from Sleep Apnea? What is the process by which your doctor determine if you are suffering from Sleep Apnea? For physicians, it is handful of tests to be performed and they've conducted research on your body's anatomy for a long time before they began their work. However, to recognize that you may have Sleep Apnea, you need to know about some indicators that will allow you to determine the most significant signs for the similar.

In the coming months, we're going to learn about the signs that may assist you in determining the cause of your body's problems.

The signs of sleep Apnea in adults

Snoring The first and most important thing to note is that Snoring is the most prominent indication of Sleep Apnea. In the majority of cases that a person having trouble sleeping, they may have Sleep Apnea. Certain people experience snoring at an older age while others experience it in a younger age. No matter what age, if you notice that someone is having trouble sleeping, have them examined because they may be suffering from Sleep Apnea.

- Sleep Apnea: You may have heard that those who suffer with Sleep Apnea have to get up at any time during the night. This is a challenge for them to remain asleep or to fall back asleep. Because of the constant waking up and falling asleep, the body doesn't have enough sleep. As a result it can cause tiredness, restlessness, and lethargy This can cause sleepiness throughout the daytime.

- Reduced Concentration Levels: It's the case that due to Sleep Apnea, your concentration levels may be affected. It is due to abrupt interruptions in your sleep pattern or sudden activation of the brain during the late hours of the night could cause problems in your memory and ability to concentrate. Not just concentration levels however, if you notice that you're experiencing sudden changes in your mood, they could also be signs that you suffer from Sleep Apnea.

The problem that is so frustrating about Sleep Apnea is that we cannot grasp the reasons behind its appearance. As a person, any like me and you would think it is a minor issue. A couple of mood swings, the inability to focus or even anything else related to these issues are seen in a different way. The mood swings should not be considered to be serious as long as they don't cause serious problems. The difficulty in concentrating is usually treated with coffee or something that contains caffeine. The key is to ensure that you comprehend, pay attention and study all symptoms and signs carefully.

Nighttime Urination: Awaking to urinate during the middle of the night is a sure sign of Sleep Apnea. This is so much that the an excessive amount of urination in the night is comparable to snoring in regards to determining whether someone suffers from Sleep Apnea. The condition is also known as Nocturnia.

What's the connection to Nocturnia as well as Sleep Apnea?

The thing that appears as Nocturnia is, in reality an outcome from a chain reaction which is caused by breath loss or the reduction in oxygen levels within the body. When the levels of oxygen decrease throughout the body blood becomes acidic, and heart rate drops. There are other problems that can be observed at the moment. It is because of all of these things that the body's body gets alert, leading to the conclusion that something is extremely wrong. The body then sends a signal to the heart regarding the excessive fluid levels. As a result, it releases an hormone that directs the body to eliminate the excess sodium and water that is within the body. This is what you could refer to as Nocturnia.

Dry Mouth: It occurs when you're not receiving enough air through your nose. You begin breathing through the mouth. Breathing in an open mouth causes dry mouth at night.

Headaches in the morning The symptom associated with Sleep Apnea is a bit unclear and not specific to this illness. However, a few patients have reported experiencing headaches in the morning. In the majority of cases headaches in the morning are an indication of OSA instead of CSA. Insufficient sleep is a major cause of headaches. In addition to this, it could be caused by fatigue or sleepiness.

-- Erectile Dysfunction There have been a variety of cases in which those suffering from OSA have Erectile dysfunction (ED). ED is the result of the reduction in the development of testosterone levels. Men naturally produce testosterone during sleep, but sleeping inability causes a decrease in testosterone production.

Sweating: It is common when you get up suddenly in the middle of the middle of the night. Additionally, it's been found that those who suffer from this disorder suffer three times as susceptible to sweating during the night than those who do not suffer from it.

High Blood Pressure Patients suffering due to Sleep Apnea may develop high blood pressure as a result. This is as a result of Sleep Apnea, blood levels become more acidic, and the blood pressure levels change abruptly. regular blood flow levels. It is important to note that elevated blood pressure can be among of the most severe signs and symptoms associated with Sleep Apnea.

Lower Stamina The capacity of a person to exercise is related to the health of their heart. If you're not able to exercise regularly it could be because your heart's condition is declining. This can cause an immediate change to how your heart operates. The exact link with Sleep Apnea and this lower stamina is still awaiting further investigation.

Depression and Anxiety It is common to connect depression to stress in the mind. However, someone with anxiety or depression may be suffering with Sleep Apnea. This is due to the fact that inability to rest well could disrupt your mental and emotional stability. It can cause anxiety and depression.

Sleep Apnea Affects Kids

Sleep Apnea is also common in children. It is also interesting that since they are still at a development stage and this condition developing at this early age is quite shocking.

Snoring: Children also snore. In many cases, they may be suffering from Obstructive Sleep Apnea. Snoring is usually seen when children sleep, you should to look for signs of snoring. Make sure to have them examined immediately after you notice this sign.

Breathing with the Mouth The children who breathe with their mouths must do it because their adenoids have grown. Because of this, airflow through their nose isn't easy. This is why they must rely on their mouths to breath properly.

Additional Symptoms other signs like insomnia and fatigue, loss of concentration, decreased focus and mood swings, as well as problems with behavior, and low academic performance share the same reasons like what you read about the adults.

In all the indications that you've read about both children and adults Snoring is the first thing you be able to observe. It is not the case when you have Obstructive Sleep Apnea. In other instances, if the snoring does not seem to be a major issue and you observe other signs that appear too often It could be that you are suffering from Central Sleep Apnea.

In the case of Complex Sleep Apnea Syndrome, research is ongoing and researchers are still studying the condition to some degree.

Whatever kind or type of Sleep Apnea you are suffering from, it is sure to affect your health. If we read on the causes and problems that result from this illness, you'll be better informed about this condition and fight it.

Chapter 20: Insomnia - How Can I Sleep?

The most commonly reported sleep disorder that is seen in the world is insomnia. It's the inability for a person to get enough sleep they need to wake in the morning feeling rejuvenated and energized to tackle the day. Many people have experienced some kind of this throughout their lives. You are awake and realize that you ought to be asleep. Dodging and turning trying to convince yourself to sleep, but fail. In the short-term, this might be just something you consumed or consumed and if it's an ongoing issue, it could be a more serious issue.

Sleepiness is often caused by depression, stress, anxiety or even the presence of a medical condition which hasn't been identified or recognized, such as hypertension or other illness. If insomnia lasts longer than two days, one must seek medical attention. This is vital since insomnia can take away the ability to perform and live your day-to-day life. However, for the majority of cases of insomnia, there are simple actions to do that can help a person get back to a regular sleep pattern.

Whatever the reason of your insomnia in the first place, becoming more at ease with your thoughts and to be able to relax will help you get a quick solution to the sleep issues. In the case of stress and anxiety, being capable of learning to relax is crucial in finding solution to this sleep disorder. There are several simple breathing exercises that will assist anyone to relax and get more restful sleep.

The practice of deep breathing can be a technique that is accessible to everyone throughout the day, and it is a relaxing tool. It's a straightforward solution that you often wonder why people aren't using it every day. It's simple to do When you're in a state of relaxation, start by breathing slowly and deeply through your diaphragm. Deep breathing brings more oxygen to your body, which helps a person physically be more comfortable and relax. It's a technique for relaxation that can be used throughout the day, especially in stressful situations, or at any time you feel anxious. It's a great habit to adopt to live a healthier life , and also for sleeping better at night.

Another more in-depth relaxation method to help you sleep is to conduct an examination of your mind and body. It involves deep breathing and engaging your imagination to concentrate on taking your body into a state of relaxation. When you breathe deep, you will be aware of how relaxing it feels throughout your body. It is recommended to start with your feet first and then move on to the anatomy while you ease into your relaxation. Be aware of the ease in your feet, then concentrate on how comfortable your ankles feel and then your calves, knees, thighs and then on until you get to your head. A lot of people struggle to get through their entire body prior to falling asleep. The mind scan helps your mind to focus on something positive rather than the anxiety and stress of the day. Keep in mind that the main reason things are better when we wake up is because we've had a restful night's rest.

If you have something happening in your life which causes anxiety or depression and causes insomnia take a step back seek out a professional to seek help. Most of the time, all you require is assistance and direction for you to return to sleep that is blissful. Some people are obstinate and do not seek assistance as it may be perceived as weakness. It is actually less important to realize you need assistance, and not seek it out. Sometimes, there are easy modifications we can implement to our diet or exercise routine which will enable the sleep cycle to be restored. It's not a great decision to try self-medicating for sleep as you've not resolved the problem, you're only trying to cover it up.

Chapter 21: Seven Steps to Stop the Insomnia Cycle Forever

These seven steps to stop the sleep cycle for good can change your life. It is crucial to ensure that each step is given the attention and focus it requires to reap the maximum benefit out of it.

These steps aren't simple fixes; they need some effort from you. When you start, stay with it. Breaking the cycle of insomnia takes change in your lifestyle and commitment.

Each stage is designed to change your perception of sleep and your sleeping. Modifying your habits is the most effective method to implement changes that stick and be an integral part of your routine. When you've completed the steps you'll start to see how transformative the process can be.

When your habits change and these habits are incorporated into your routine, sleepiness becomes something you can modify, instead of something that you struggle to deal with.

Sleepiness is more prevalent in women than males. Everybody responds to the your circadian rhythm. The circadian rhythm determines your sleep and wake cycle. It is tuned to the cycles of light and dark in the natural world. If your circadian rhythm is not in time, you'll suffer from insomnia.

Sleeping disorders can be short-term or prolonged, and both of which respond to modifications and the steps described included in this section. Keep in mind that these steps are intended to assist you in changing your habits and beliefs about sleep. The way you are thinking about sleep, about the place you sleep and the routine you adhere to throughout the day will have an impression on your daily life and will break the cycle of insomnia.

Step 1

Regularly scheduled sleep and wake up Time

I can imagine what you're thinking,"how can I get regular sleeping and waking times if I am suffering from an insomnia-like condition?" There is a solution.

The act of slapping your fingers and announcing the time you'll go to sleep and when you will awake isn't going to make any difference; changing the way you think about sleeping can.

Incredibly, our thoughts can alter our thinking and behave. Setting a time when you go to bed and when to rise will help you reset your circadian rhythm and get you get ready to meet the Sandman.

Set a time for going to bed to give you at minimum 8 hours of sleep before you get up in the morning to go to work.

The time you choose to set is symbolic and also an instruction for your mind to pay attention to. When you've found a sleeping time that you are comfortable with, you can set an appropriate wake-up time.

When you are deciding to wake up at a certain time consider the amount of time you will need.

You would like to relax before you leave to work. Allow yourself plenty of time to get up and get your day started without getting caught up in the rush or feeling with stress.

Your time of wake and sleep must be considered essential elements of your routine. they are just as crucial to your well-being as your meals and the work you do at school or at work. You should put your best effort to these times that you've chosen and then you should remind yourself of how crucial they are.

These positive thoughts about sleep and waking up will eventually become part of your mind and aid you battle insomnia.

Take a look at it this way you've probably got an estimated time when you can go to bed and that is likely to stress you out because you are aware that you're not going to sleep or have brought work home and you're stressed about finishing the task before going to bed.

You may also be battling an array of negative thoughts and feelings regarding getting up. You worry about not hearing the alarm, or not sleeping enough prior to the alarm going off...the list goes on and on.

All these negative thoughts about falling asleep and waking up have impressions on the mind and, eventually, the rhythm of your circadian cycle.

Then, pick two great timings, that will allow you to enjoy a full 8 hours of rest and allow you to rise and begin your day with ease, without any stress!

Do not worry about things that affect your sleeping time or morning wake-up time. It might be difficult initially, but eventually things will settle down.

The next step is to assist you in sticking to your set time of wake and sleep without causing anxiety or anxiety.

Step 2

Get ready for sleep

This is an essential stage, getting ready for sleep will soon become routine, and routines are the behaviors that allow you to accomplish things in the manner you would like to get them done.

It is a process of repetition. Repeated behavior turns into habit, and the process of becoming habits open the doorway to changes in behavior that could improve your life and your objectives or not.

The key is that you will take control of your conduct and the outcomes No more wishful thinking or whining, it's time to act.

The process of preparing for sleep is to create an routine that allows you to feel relaxed, tired, and get to bed ready to go asleep. Your routine should include positive emotions, thoughts, and relationships that will make you feel relaxed and ready to drift off to sleep.

This routine of preparation will alter your thoughts about how you go to bed, and how you feel once you finally get to your bed.

Write down the things you love to do to can help you relax. It could be reading a book an aromatic bath and meditation or even a pastime you like. When you've made your list, record the way you feel each time you consider these relaxing things.

Note in your journal your thoughts as well as feelings alongside the things that make you relax. Make sure you set aside at least an hour to engage in one of these activities each at night prior to going to bed.

The hour you've reserved is likely the most important shift you'll make. When the time comes to unwind and relax in your personal time before bed, do not let anything get in your way.

You should write about the way this activity calms you and provides you with a tranquil time during the day. Do not forget the section about writing down your thoughts It is crucial to reinforce positive feelings and positive thoughts associated with this type of activity. The next step will help support this process and assist you to adhere to the plan.

Step 3.

Create Your Bedroom to be a sleeping Paradise

The place you sleep in can alter your sleeping habits. Create an area that is devoted to sleeping only (and sexual activity of course!). The bedroom should not have a TV This may be difficult to reconcile but you can't have television watching while you sleep.

This list will assist you to make your dream bed:

There was no television in the room.

There's no PC in this room

Decorate using soothing shades, no distractions or stimulating

Be attentive to the patterns, textures, colors and patterns in your bedroom.

Make sure the room is cool. It's more comfortable to sleep in cool temperatures.

It is essential not to be watching television or play on your computer in the bedroom. In the dark room while you sleep. Light could affect your naturally occurring circadian rhythm. If the room is lit from street lights, neighbors or road lights consider using darkening curtains or shades to prevent light from disrupting your sleep.

Artificial light, particularly blue light, the type of light from computers and televisions can disrupt the production of melatonin. Melatonin hormone is involved in the regulation of sleep. Glasses with a tint of amber have been found to reduce the amount of blue light that is emitted to your eyes. Wearing these glasses in the evening before going to going to bed could cut down on the quantity of blue light that enters your eyes and stop it from reducing production of melatonin.

Cooling the room can assist you in falling to sleep. As your body starts to prepare itself to sleep, it starts in releasing warmth from its body's core, which is then released to the skin and the outside. If the environment is too hot, the process takes longer to complete and can cause sleepiness.

Step 4

Fitness and Nature Light

Incorporate a fitness routine into your routine. In the event that you have a workout routine or are beginning one, be sure you are taking some exercise place outside.

Natural sunlight throughout the day will aid in regulating your circadian cycle.

Exercise can help you sleep in the night. The more physical activity and sunshine you can get at night, the greater chances you'll have of getting a good night's sleep.

The circadian rhythm of your body is an intricate one making sure you get the right amount of light and darkness will regulate your inner clock, which will allow sleep and remain in a deep sleep.

One of the most effective method for resetting your circadian rhythm is going camping. Camping and exposure to the natural daylight and dark hours can reset your internal clock, and help you get back to sleep every night.

Step 5

Diet Changes

There's no need to alter anything about your diet in order to ease sleepiness. Incorporating some carbs into your dinner can assist you in falling asleep. Carbs release tryptophan, which helps induce sleep.

If you're following the low carb diet and you are sleeping less, it is possible that your diet is contributing to your sleepiness.

It's not a good idea to consume large quantities of food prior to bedtime or drink a lot of alcohol prior to the bed. Take a minimum of 4 hours before going to bed so that your body has the time to digest food before you fall asleep.

Incorporating carbs into your final meal will slowly release tryptophan through your system. By the time you're in sleeping, you'll feel naturallly asleep.

Avoid eating carb-rich food before going to bed. take it in between your final meal, to give the carbs the chance to breakdown and assist you to fall asleep.

Alcohol is a solution that everybody talks about, however it's not a solution in fact, it's the cause of. Alcohol consumption before bed can make you sleep better than you would normally, but it could also make you wake up.

Alcohol can make you feel energetic and make you wake up at night. This is not the best way to have an uninterrupted sleep. Remove alcohol and include some carbs. This will allow you to sleep better and remain asleep.

Step 6

No More Stimulants

Eliminate any stimulants in your diet. It might be difficult but it will help improve your sleeping. Don't drink any coffee or decaf coffee. Coffee regardless of what time of the day you consume it, could cause adverse effects on your sleep. The effects of caffeine are long-lasting in the body and can cause a lot of trouble when it comes to sleep.

Caffeine is present in more than coffee. It is also found in cola drinks and other soft drinks, so make sure you be sure to read the labels. It can be found in all kinds of tea except when it is decaffeinated and beware of chocolate. Chocolate has caffeine as well.

Eliminating stimulants from your food can help you return to the natural cycle of sleep and wake. This will not occur overnight but it will happen. Follow the methods to remove the intake of stimulants and your naturally recurring sleep cycles will occur. Replace the drinks of caffeine with water. it is vital to keep our bodies in balance, and dehydration may creep up on you and lead to leg cramps which is another cause of sleep loss.

Step 7

If You Don't Go Sleep, Make Yourself Up

If you do these steps, you'll begin to see the normal sleep cycle returning. When you're implementing the steps above, this one is crucial.

If you don't get to sleep within half hour, take a break. It may be counterintuitive to someone suffering from insomnia however, you'll find that it can help.

If you are unable to sleep and get out of the room. If you are in bed, and you try to make yourself sleepy can only lead to anger and will stimulate your mind and thoughts. It is much better to take a step forward.

Try moving to a different space and reading the book which is not a digital one or a normal book. Digital books emit blue light. This light can be stimulating. Take a break and read a magazine or a book or anything else that soothes you and doesn't make you feel awake.

When you start feeling tired Return to your bedroom and attempt to go to sleep.

If All else fails

The methods in this guide will restore your natural circadian rhythm , and you'll once more get a good night's rest. If these steps don't function as expected then there's a second option such as seeking cognitive therapy.

Cognitive therapy addresses the reasons that you are unable to fall asleep. Sometimes , there are reasons why that make it difficult to sleep, and when stress keeps you awake, despite your best efforts Cognitive therapists can help you.

Cognitive therapy is all about understanding and applying behavioral techniques to aid you in overcoming sleeplessness. The methods of this guide are similar to the techniques used in behavioral therapy, however having a relationship with a counselor is one step ahead. It is possible to overcome, and if you require some assistance to relax you, a cognitive counselor can assist.

Another major factor that affects those who suffer from insomnia is their health. Be aware that health issues can trigger insomnia. Certain medicines can trigger insomnia. In this book, make sure there aren't any underlying medical issues that may be the cause of your sleepiness.

Chapter 22: The Things You Need to Learn about Sleep Aids for Prescription

Before you start taking any prescribed sleep aids, it's advised to consult your physician about the risks involved in taking medications prescribed by a doctor. The doctors recommend that certain sleep aids shouldn't be used for more than 2 weeks. Be aware that with any prescription medications you use, there might be negative side effects. Also, when taken for a long time it could lead to an addiction to those prescription medications.

Here are some tips to take certain receptors in order to get an improved night's rest.

Hypnotics (Lunesta and Ambian)

Lunesta is an sedative as well as hypnotic medication that is not recommended for children. Like any prescription drug it is possible to experience dangerous negative side negative effects.

Here's a list of possible adverse effects:

Confusion

Depression

Aggression

Memory issues

Anxiety

Agitation

Hallucinations

Day-time drowsiness

Feeling hungover

Dry mouth

Frequent dizzy spells

Lunesta (also also known as eszopiclone) is an effective medication for insomnia. It is administered by labs and other outpatient departments. It is prescribed at bedtime. The dose that is the lowest is 1 mg, however it can be increased up to 2mg or

3mg if a physician feels that this is necessary.

For older people doses is not to exceed 2 mg.

Ambien

Ambien (also also known as Zolpidem) is an medicine for adults suffering from sleep issues. It aids in getting sleep faster and helps the brain relax to induce a peaceful mental state.

The medicine usually is accompanied by written instructions on how to use it and when and what the recommended dosage amounts must be. This information is supplied by your pharmacist when you get the prescription. It's always recommended to consult your physician and pharmacist questions regarding the dangers and adverse effects of a medication.

This medicine is taken orally after eating, and typically at the night. It's very effective and is best taken prior to going to getting to bed. Don't operate any machines, drive, or engage in any activity in which you have to be alert following the use of it.

Consult an experienced physician if you are experiencing withdrawal symptoms or other reactions that make you feel sick.

It's not advisable to consume a significant dose of this drug if have a history of substance abuse as it could lose its effectiveness.

Here's a list of possible adverse effects:

Dizziness

Memory loss

Hallucinations

Suicidal thoughts

Depression

Confusion

Aggression

Anxiety

Dual Orexin Receptor Antagonists (Belsomra)

Belsomra is a selective antagonist of Orexin receptors that treat insomnia. There are some side effects of this medication as well.

Here's a list of possible the side effects:

Headaches

Sleepiness

Abnormal dreams

Diarrhea

Dry mouth

Dry cough

Infections of the chest

Drool

The serious adverse effects include sleepwalking, as well as other activities that you would not normally do during sleep.

Additionally, it doesn't react well with alcohol, grapefruit juiceor antibiotics, and anti-fungals. It is recommended to tell your physician about all supplements or medications you're taking to ensure that you are in the best possible position. It is also advised not to be used during pregnancy except when prescribed by your doctor. Also, you should consult your doctor prior to breastfeeding when you intend to take this medication.

Anxiolytics of the Melatonin Receptor (Rozerem)

The sedative and hypnotic medication is a drug that affects specific chemicals in your body. They then regulate your sleep cycles.

Rozerem is frequently utilized to treat insomnia and could be the least addictive of sleep medication. It is not at risk of dependence, and you should not use this medication in the event of sleep apnea. Also, you is not recommended when you suffer from breathing disorders or any other type.

This medication can trigger an extremely severe allergic reaction. If you have an adverse reaction, talk your doctor or seek urgent medical attention. There are some side effects of this medication.

Here's a list of possible adverse effects:

Face swelling

Your mouth may become distorted

Your tongue could become larger

Your throat could be blocked

Vomiting

Hives

Nausea

Anti-Depressants (Silenor)

Silenor (otherwise known as the doxepin) is an anti-depressant medication utilized to treat sleep issues. But, be aware that using this medication as an sedative may cause additional problems. Talk to your doctor in case you experience any negative side effects for example:

Drool

Nausea

Vomiting

Diarrhea

Constipation

Insanity and imbalance

Numbness

Feeling tingly

The dosage recommended for Silenor is 6mg every day. It is not recommended to take it right after eating and shouldn't be taken in conjunction with alcohol. Silenor can also trigger mild depression. It could cause death if given to someone who is already suicidal. Be conscious of this prior to making an appointment to receive this medication.

Chapter 23: Lifestyle Changes

Alongside stress reduction and a healthy diet your sleeping routine can be improved with small lifestyle changes. They are not large-scale changes that can be integrated into your daily routine, but they require little effort by your side. These are:

Make your bed transform:

Your bed should be a space where you are free to spread out and uncluttered of clutter or distractions that could affect your sleep negatively. Remove any unnecessary clutter that's placed on or near your mattress. Laptop, trailing wires, fancy cushions, etc. are only some examples. You should try to find the right mattress for your back. This is particularly important for those older than 40, as the wrong mattress can cause back pain, too.

Here are a few suggestions to manage noise in your bedroom:

- Use earplugs.

Install double-parred windows. embellish with curtains that are heavy,

Make use of a fan or device which produces steady "white sound". The devices that produce white noise are offered on the market to remove all other disturbances.

Dim the lighting in the area:

In order to enjoy the most optimal quality sleep, you should try to block any light sources in your bedroom. Switch off all devices with LEDs into them. Also, make sure that the curtains are properly covering the windows, if you intend to sleep later.

Researchers from the Max Planck Institute have found by conducting a series of studies that when individuals were kept in a closed environment , and then told to rest their circadian rhythms reacted to a more consistent pattern. The changes in the intensity of light in the room demonstrated that the patterns changed when light intensity increased. Light intensity was in direct correlation to production of Melatonin the hormone responsible for sleep.

Eliminate Blue Light:

It is the spectrum which is comprised of seven colors. There is a variety in frequencies (energy) which are released from any light source. Of all the wavelengths, red light is the one with the lowest amount of energy, while blue light is the highest energy. You may have noticed the fact that using a smartphone or laptop prior to going to bed can disrupt sleep patterns. The sleepiness gradually fades and , before you know it you've been spending the entire evening surfing the web.

The primary reason for this lies in the presence of blue light which can decrease melatonin production dramatically dropping to 39 percent. Even if you are planning to install a tiny night-time bulb, not use a bulb that emits blue light.

Conclusion

I hope that this book has been useful in recognizing that the most simple way to go about your world is pull the covers to cover your face and head to bed. Also, I hope this book can provide the answers to all possible questions about sleeping.

We have made every effort to show in this book that sleep can make people more relaxed and less anxious, awake, or simply happy, whether in the outside or within your own. One simple message given is that if a thriving nation were to focus on getting more rest, it would result in a happier and more assured group of people. That is the greatest accomplishment of humanity. We certainly expect our devoted readers to be more educated about the fact that it's an everyday occurrence that a challenge that is difficult to solve at night can be solved in the morning , after the sleep committee has been working on the issue. I hope that this book can find an avenue to your bed prior to a Good Night Sleep! !

It is now time to put into practice the information you've learned from this book. If you do not apply the concepts you've learned, knowledge is useless! The best-selling and internationally recognized writer, Tony Robbins often says "Knowledge alone isn't enough. You have to act it isn't just through learning new knowledge that our lives will improve by taking on new actions. Therefore, I urge you from the bottom of my soul to act on the lessons you've learned from this book and, I'm sure you'll find that the only issue you'll face is that you didn't get this book six months ago and act immediately!

Thanks for your kind words and good luck!

www.ingramcontent.com/pod-product-compliance
Lightning Source LLC
Chambersburg PA
CBHW060331030426
42336CB00011B/1297